The Emu Farmer's Handbook

Phillip Minnaar and Maria Minnaar

NYONI
PUBLISHING CO.
GROVETON, TEXAS

First Published by
INDUNA COMPANY

Illustrations by Maria Minnaar
Photographs by Phillip and Maria Minnaar

Sixth Printing: October. 1995

ISBN 0-9643741-1-0 Printed in U.S.A.

INDEX

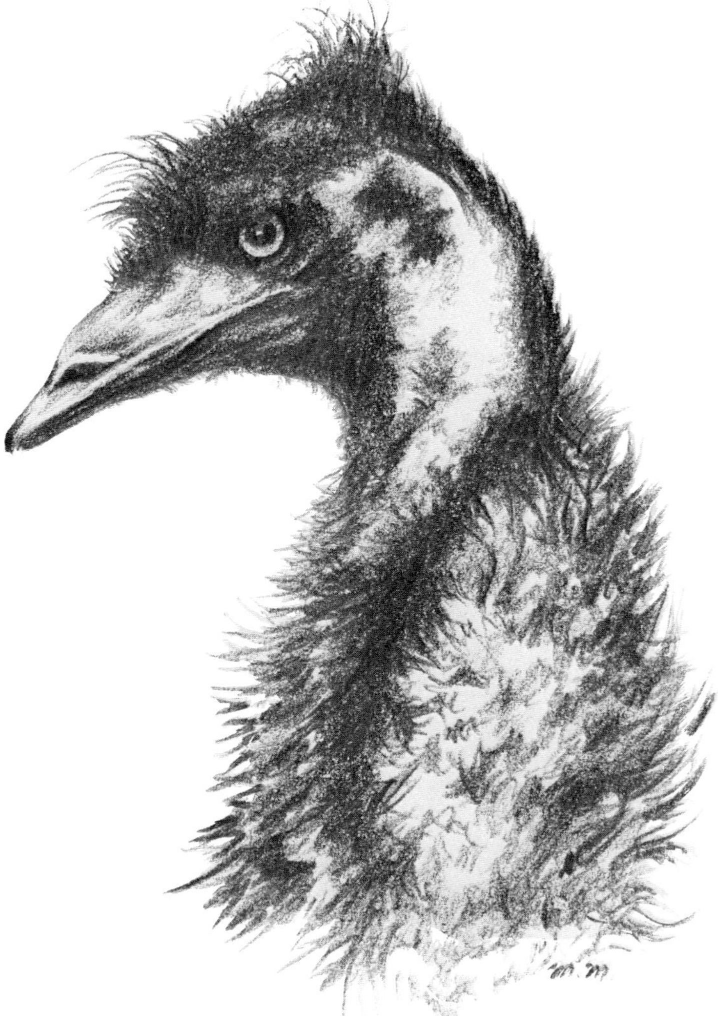

CHAPTER 1

An Introduction to Commercial Emu Farming

Successful farming of the emu must be based on sound management practices in incubation, hatching, nutrition, record keeping and overall operations.

1.1 EMU - GENERAL INFORMATION

• Native to Australia.

• Belongs to the Ratite family of flightless birds, which also includes the Ostrich (Africa), Rhea (South America), Cassowary (Australia and New Guinea) and Kiwi (New Zealand).

• Found in significant numbers in the United States - offspring of birds originally imported some decades ago for zoos/collections - now farmed here as alternative livestock.

• Productive (average of 30 to 40 eggs per year from mature breeding pair when eggs are continually removed for artificial incubation)

• Long-lived (up to 30 years recorded by zoos)

• Temperament: generally docile, occasionally fight among themselves. Curious.

• Adaptable to most climatic conditions.

• Size: 5 to 6 foot, weigh up to 150 lbs. when mature. Attain full height by about a year.

• Breeding age: between 2 and 3 years old.

• Three color stages during growth:

1. Hatch to about 2 months: Longitudinally striped.
2. 3 months to about 1 year: Uniform chocolate brown/beige with head and neck darker.
3. Mature birds: Bare blue neck outlined with black feathers, mottled body feather coloration. No color differences between males and females.

1.2 COMMERCIAL EMU FARMING

Emu farming in the United States does not as yet have a long history behind it. In mid-1989 a national association was started in Texas by emu farmers, with the idea to promote, improve and research emu farming as a serious alternative type of livestock.

Emus are easily domesticated and emu farming is a low-overhead business. The feed costs per bird are minimal as are land and labor requirements for the bird, in spite of its large size. Emus are also very productive, giving multiple offspring every season.

Very little information about emu farming has been available to date, because this type of farming had never been done before except on a small scale as an aboriginal project in Western Australia. This handbook is the result of several years of research done to help the emu farmer understand more about the emu and how it works.

In Australia, the emu has for hundreds of years been regarded as little more than a pest. Many were hunted down and slaughtered in the past, in order to try and control the large flocks that migrated across Western Australia at certain times of the year, trampling and destroying many farmers' entire crop harvests as they went. Eventually, several hundred miles of "emu-proof" fencing was erected across much of Western Australia to keep the birds out of the crop-farming areas. Culling (by game rangers) still takes place to keep numbers constant, but harvesting of emus in the wild by individuals is not allowed and carries stiff penalties. Only the Aborigines are allowed to hunt emu, and may only kill what they need to eat. No selling of by-products such as the leather, etc. is permitted in these cases. In recent years, however, the commercial value of the emu has begun to receive some recognition in Western Australia, and as a result, a small number of farmers there have received permission to raise the birds for commercial purposes. Initially, only two of the emu's products - the leather and the oil - were considered marketable, with carved eggs and feathers being a small sideline. Most Australians did not even consider the meat as having any potential, as it was rumored to be very oily. However, several emu farmers in the United States tried it and found it to be delicious, with an appearance and taste very similar to beef and a fat content about the same as turkey (according to several laboratory analyses that have been done). Probably, the rumors about "oily meat" came from incorrect slaughtering. If the layer of fat is not removed prior to cutting the meat from the bird, it might indeed get on the meat and make it oily.

Emu fat, or the oil rendered from it, has been used for many centuries by the Aborigines to soothe the pains of arthritis, and as an emollient for dry skin. Emu oil has a deep penetrating quality, will keep for extended periods of time, without becoming rancid, and is readily miscible with other substances. More research needs to be done in order to assess fully its actual medicinal potential, but as far as skin creams/ cosmetics goes, the Australians have already developed and are marketing a moisturizing cream using emu oil as its base. Research is currently underway to develop formulas for skin creams here in the U.S. also.

Emu leather is another of the products of this very versatile bird and is in demand on the European fashion market. The fine-grained emu hide is similar to ostrich in appearance but with quill-marks less prominent and closer together, giving it an attractive rippling appearance. It is also much thinner and softer than ostrich leather, making it more suitable for the fashion garment industry than the boot-making business.

Some people may be concerned about the future of the emu as a species if it is farmed commercially, especially for slaughter. As an emu farmer and also as a believer in wildlife/nature conservation, I feel that farming the emu poses no threat at all to its future survival, but quite the opposite. Firstly, even though there is a sizeable population of emus in the United States at the moment, it is not native to this country and therefore will only be found here in a domesticated or semi-domesticated situation, and not running wild. "Conservation" of emus is therefore not really an issue here in the U.S. Secondly, in Australia, the emu's country of origin, such stringent conservation laws are in effect (as well as a ban on the export of live emus or fertile eggs), that its survival in the wild is ensured. Thirdly, the successful domestication of any animal automatically ensures not only its survival, but the improvement of the species as well, by means of selective breeding. Domestication, with the ultimate goal of using an animal's products, has in fact been known to save some species from extinction - a good example being the American buffalo.

The emu, in conclusion, is a tough bird that does not easily succumb to disease. For all its size, it is also a docile bird which is relatively easily handled and does not generally show any aggression to humans, even in the breeding season.

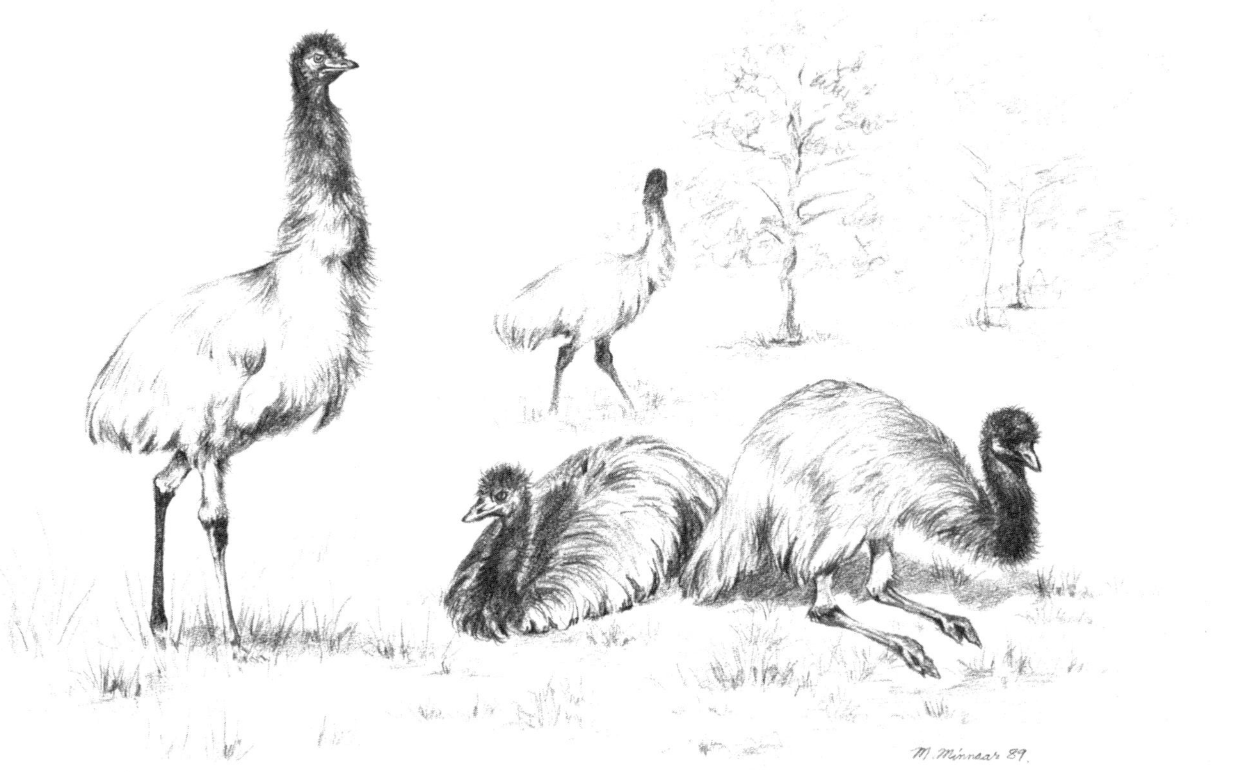

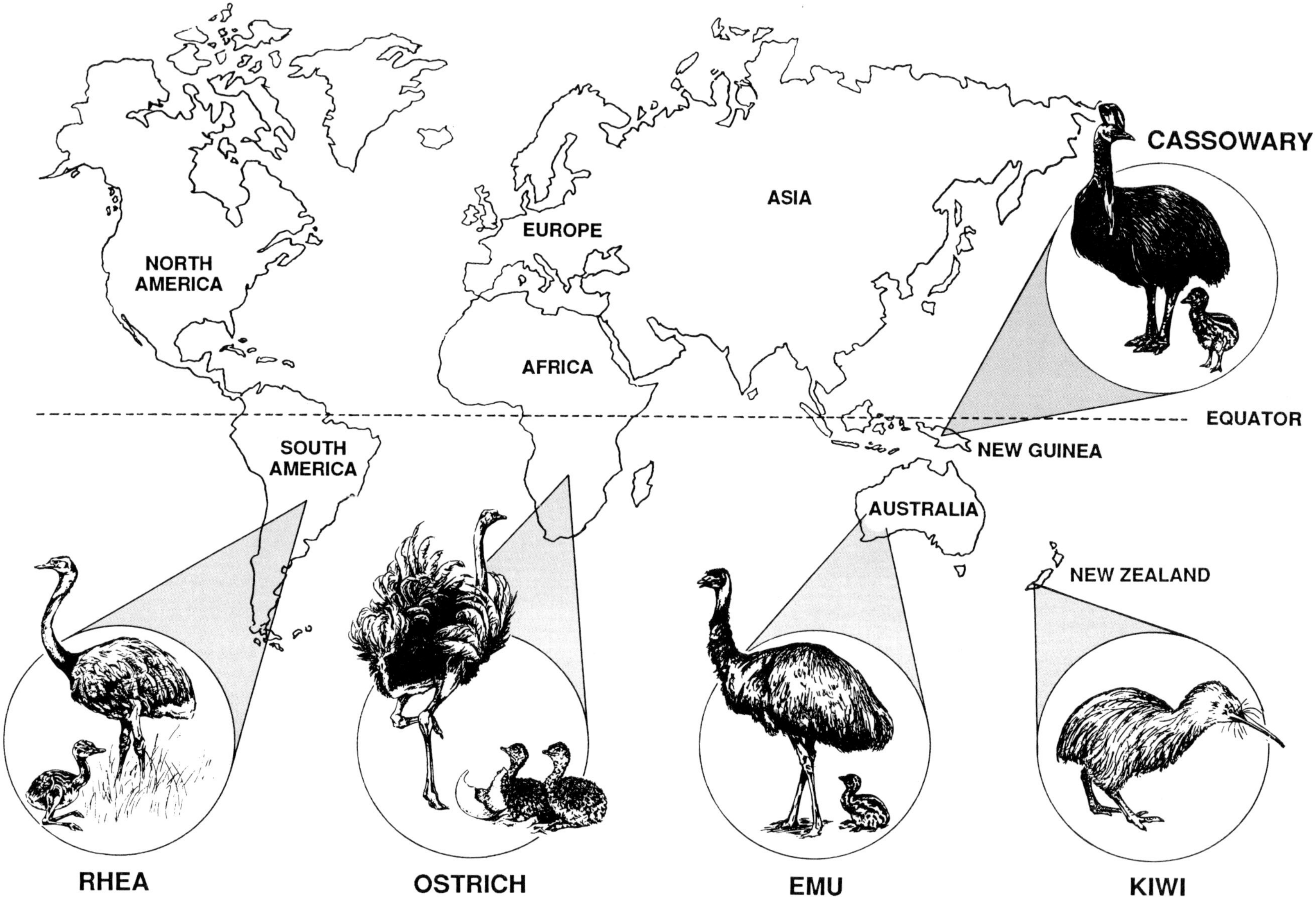

Fig 1.1 - Map showing natural distribution of ratites throughout the world.

CHAPTER 2

Farm Management

The farmer, who produces food/fiber products for the use of his fellow man, has a very important responsibility: to manage his land wisely so that it will continue to yield a good crop of plants or animals for food and other necessary products.

There are risks associated with any type of livestock farming. Some losses due to accidents, illnesses or reproductive failure are inevitable. However, by the use of good management practices, many problems can be avoided and good overall production will result.

2.1 GOOD MANAGEMENT

The factors involved in good management of any emu farming operation are:

- SELECTION OF GOOD STOCK - For the novice emu farmer, the second opinion of an experienced person can be of benefit, whether he buys birds from an auction or from another breeder.

- CONTENTED BIRDS - Providing an environment that is as efficient and stress-free for the birds as possible makes good farming sense. This also means caring for the birds adequately by providing good nutrition, good sanitation and shelter from the elements. A daily routine is also helpful in minimizing stress.

- OVERALL CLEANLINESS - While no farm can be germ-free, factors such as not overcrowding pens, making sure there is good drainage and keeping shelters and feeders reasonably clean are good sanitation practices which will minimize the spread of disease. Extra care should be taken to keep the incubator room clean, of course, including restricting visitors during breeding season and removal of dirty footwear before entering.

- GOOD "EYE" FOR BIRDS - The ability to spot problems in birds is something that develops with experience and through keen daily observation. The earlier a problem can be detected, the quicker it can be cured. Prompt action often means fewer losses.

- GOOD OVERALL KNOWLEDGE OF EMUS - This is the reason for this book. The more you know, the better equipped you are to deal with any situation.

- COMMON SENSE.

2.2 BIRD SELECTION

The selection of birds to be used for breeding purposes, whether they are adults, yearlings or chicks at time of purchase, is a very important part of farming emus.

Basic livestock farming principles should be adhered to, as follows:

(a) Physical soundness and general good health

Check for the following:

- Knock-knees or splayed legs, especially in chicks
- Curvature of the spine or neck
- Eye infections
- Dull feathers, emaciation, other signs of illness
- Excessively wild birds - prone to injury
- Blood in stool, which indicates problems (check stool in pens)
- Extremely dome-shaped back
- Obesity

To check for deviations, watch the bird walk and run directly from the front and directly from the back. Legs that flail outward or a neck that is off-center should be readily apparent. It is hard to detect small deviations in the vertebrae of very fat birds, so these should be caught and felt along the backbone. While a lot of extra fat may be desirable for slaughter birds, it is undesirable in potential breeders. An excessive amount of fat is when you can feel a layer thicker than about ½" on top of the ribs, by the sternum and under the wings. Emus have hardly any breast meat, so if there is a thick fat layer it can easily be felt in those places.

(b) Sexing

Make sure the sexes are correct, and that the conditions of sale are understood.

(c) Selection of seller

Select birds from emu farmers that have progressive breeding plans. Good emu farmers should be working towards establishing better bloodlines by selecting birds with desirable traits that they have hatched themselves, to place in the breeder program. Pairs that are already producing and that are the result of such selections are the marks of a good, well-established emu farmer. The operation itself should also show good management overall.

(d) Unrelated birds

For good foundation stock, try to get unrelated birds. Line-breeding (inbreeding) is a controversial subject. The idea behind line-breeding is to perpetuate desirable characteristics. Birds that are conformationally correct should produce correct offspring, with all or most of the good features prominent in the offspring, even if the birds are related. However, this may be something to strive for later, after it has been established which particular good characteristics one would like to breed for. High egg production (with good hatchability) is certainly something to strive for. In the beginning, however, it is good to have the genetic variety of unrelated birds, and it will certainly do no harm.

(e) Preparation

Get the advice of one or more experienced emu farmers, and take time to see different farms and options before buying. Plan ahead, prepare a budget and learn all you can - in other words, do your "homework" before bringing home the birds.

2.3 PENS AND FACILITIES

There are many different ways to farm emus and most of them work well. However, some work better for larger groups of birds, or the climate or type of land may have an effect on how best to lay out your pens. This chapter will give some suggestions and reasons for doing things, and emu farmers may draw from this information to design their farms in the most suitable way.

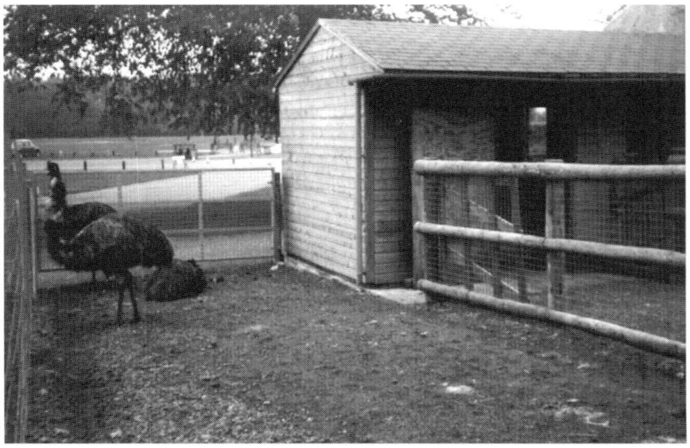

Plate 2.1 - Emu enclosure in England, with wooden shelter.

Emus are naturally used to open spaces and they are nomadic birds, so by nature they are not used to confinement. This means that contrary to some beliefs, there is no such thing as an "ideal pen size", since any type of confinement actually deviates from the natural conditions. However, emus do adapt very well and have been kept for extended periods in areas as small as 10' x 10' (in barns or stalls) during very harsh, cold periods of winter, and have continued to produce many fertile eggs even under these conditions. Commercial emu farming will probably lean more towards smaller pens during laying season for better labor efficiency (feeding, collecting eggs etc.) On the other hand, on some ranches emus have been free to roam in 200-acre enclosures and have produced many fertile eggs under those conditions also. Nevertheless, both these situations are ones of confinement, and some emus will need time to adapt to either.

If breeder birds are to be kept in small breeder pens as illustrated in **Fig. 2.1(b)**, it is recommended to have a turnout area where birds can run for about 1 to 3 months in the off-season to exercise and mingle with other birds. Any aggressive birds will need to be separated from the more docile emus, but generally if the pen is large enough and contains some trees and brush, the aggressor will give up the chase once the bird(s) he/she is chasing are concealed behind some such visual barrier.

Before and during breeding season, young potential first-time breeders in particular need to be watched if paired up randomly and placed in small breeding pens. They should be split up immediately if they start to fight. By watching and acting quickly, serious emu farmers rarely have this problem get out of hand. The birds may be separated temporarily by using welded-wire panels (e.g. cattle panels) to split the pen in half until they start eating together at the dividing panel without one threatening the other.

Generally, these problems can take place in pens from 10' x 10' up to about 50' x 100', with the danger of injury obviously being greater (as it can take place quicker) in the smaller pen. If the young birds are paired correctly, however (see **Section 7.2**), this problem rarely occurs.

Alleys between pens are handy to move birds along when changing pens, to load birds from when they are being taken to a new location, and to place a bird in if he needs to be separated and there is no spare pen available. The use of alleys in pairing young birds is described in **Section 7.2**. Alleys also provide easy access for feeding and collecting eggs, and provide a "safety net" in case a gate is left open and a bird escapes from its pen.

Shelters

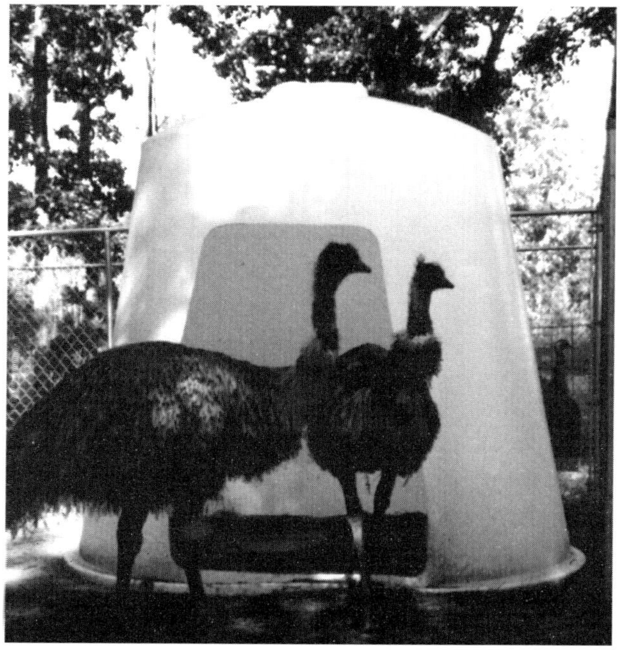

Plate 2.2 - Molded-plastic shelter for emu breeder pair.

While it is important to have trees and other vegetation in pens for shade, shelter, and to give the birds a more natural situation, a shelter to lay eggs in is also a good idea. In wet climates it is a necessity, as hatchability is poor from wet and muddy eggs. Shelters do not need to be especially big or elaborate: a three-sided, roofed wood-and-metal structure is used by some emu farmers, and a more portable molded plastic or greenhouse-type structure by others. **Plate 2.2** shows a molded plastic shelter, which is actually a converted grain silo. (A hole for an opening was cut into the side.) The types of shelter which allow light in have the added advantage of being more appealing to the birds than a shelter in which they cannot see well, and are also less likely to promote growth of molds, bacteria and other harmful organisms which prefer dark places. Clean hay or straw is ideal bedding for these shelters, and should encourage nest-making/egg-laying inside the shelters, besides providing a warm, dry and comfortable place to sleep. The hay should be changed regularly to ensure clean, dry laying conditions.

Drainage

Good drainage of the pens is very important, not only for hygienic reasons but also because any puddles that form at the fence tend to become trenches as the emus pace back and forth in them, walking the fence-line.

Rugged terrain and sloping land is no problem for most emus. Fence-building, feeding and egg-collecting may be a little more difficult in such situations, but for the farmer who wants to utilize barren, rocky land on which few other types of livestock can be raised, placing his emus there may be just the answer.

Fencing

A mesh-wire fence such as chainlink or horse-wire provide the ideal type of fencing for the serious emu farmer. A fence made of wire strands is very easy for an emu to get out of, and barbed wire should never be used in conjunction with other fencing since emus tend to rub along the fence and could injure themselves. The height should be 5½' to 6', preferably with a top rail for greater strength and support. Thinner posts such as chainlink pipe or T-posts are recommended. Large wooden posts along fences are often run into by emus, causing injury, especially among young (more skittish) birds. If wooden posts are used, they should be on the outside of the fence to minimize this danger. Turn all wire fasteners outwards so as not to scrape or injure a bird's neck.

Chick facilities

Many different facilities for raising chicks work well, with the size of the operation (number of chicks) being a major factor in choosing the right design. The most important factors to consider are:

1. Number of birds
2. Hygiene
3. Cost of facility
4. Efficiency

Small farmers can keep their chicks inside in clean cardboard boxes with hay and sometimes a small towel for bedding for the first week, allowing them out during the day if weather permits. When they are old enough to go into a bigger pen, the box can be discarded or burnt and a new one used for the next batch of chicks. No more than ten chicks should sleep together in a box, and warmth is important as cold chicks huddle up very close and the risk of smothering is increased. This is a very easy and hygienic way to raise chicks, but it is impractical to do with large amounts of birds.

Larger operations will have an indoor chick sleeping area, compartmented as needed, with an outdoor run attached. The floor inside can be concrete, but not smooth, or the chicks will slip. The chicks can go out during the day while the inside is hosed clean. A slight incline in the floor makes for easier cleaning. A disinfectant used in washing the floor will help keep bacterial infections and molds (fungi) in check. The floors may or may not be heated, depending on the climate and the age of chicks (younger chicks needing more warmth.) For those unwilling to go to the expense of heated flooring, there are heating mats available on the market on which chicks can sleep, and of course heat lamps can also be used to add warmth from above. Alternately, the floor may be covered with outdoor type carpet, as long as the carpet is regularly washed and replaced with a clean dry one. Another alternative is to cover the indoor run with a large sheet of plastic, then a layer of wood shavings to absorb moisture, followed by a layer of clean hay. The birds can run around easily on the hay, do not generally eat it and can sleep comfortably on it. Hay should be turned daily so droppings go down into the wood shavings, and should be changed frequently. When the birds are large enough or the weather warm enough to make the hay no longer necessary, the plastic, shavings and hay can all be rolled up and discarded easily. This method also works well if temporary chick pens have to be set up inside a barn or other building. One- to two-foot-high pens can be quickly made by bolting together some sheets of plywood or other board for sides, and spreading plastic sheeting/shavings/hay for the bottom. When the pens are no longer needed, the side panels can be unbolted and stacked against a wall where they will be out of the way.

Dirt floors in the inside runs also work fairly well, but cleanup is harder. An alternative is to have outside chick runs where each run has its own portable plastic/fiberglass shelter, which has no bottom and can be moved periodically to another area in the pen to allow the sun and elements to kill any harmful organisms that have started growing inside. Hay may be placed in these shelters for additional insulation, and heat lamps can also be used. This reduces the need for a large indoor chick facility.

In any type of design chosen, it is important to remember that the easier a facility is to keep clean, the more likely you are to keep it clean. The cleaner the facility, the healthier the chicks. Therefore it is in the interests of good production as well as time- and labor- efficiency to make everything as easy for yourself as possible.

From about 2 to 3 months, chicks can stay in larger groups of 20 to 40 as long as it is not too cold as this will cause them to "huddle" together, increasing risks of smothering. Chicks do best with a lot of room to exercise, in pens at least 50' x 100'. It is still important to keep chicks together that are close in age and in size, so that larger chicks do not crowd out smaller ones from feeders, or peck and harass them. Lining the bottom part of the fence with a small-mesh wire (e.g. chicken wire) will prevent smaller chicks from getting out of the pens. Spring-loaded gates are also a good idea to prevent escape.

Rotation

Because emu farming is intensive, pens sometimes get trampled completely bare of vegetation. Not only does manure then lie on the ground longer instead of being utilized by growing plants, but also, concentrations of bacteria or parasites or other harmful organisms can become greater in certain places, especially areas which remain dark, warm and damp for extended periods. The fact that most emus spend most of their lives in outside rather than inside facilities probably minimizes the spread of

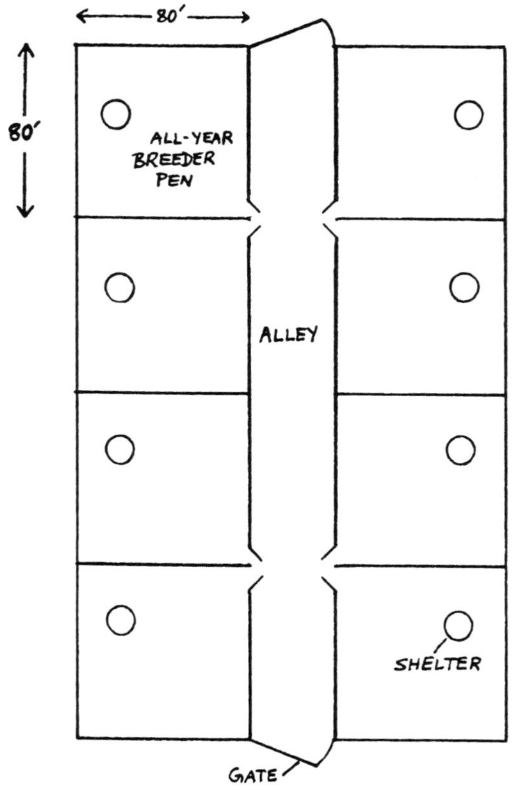

Fig. 2.1(a) All-year breeder pens.

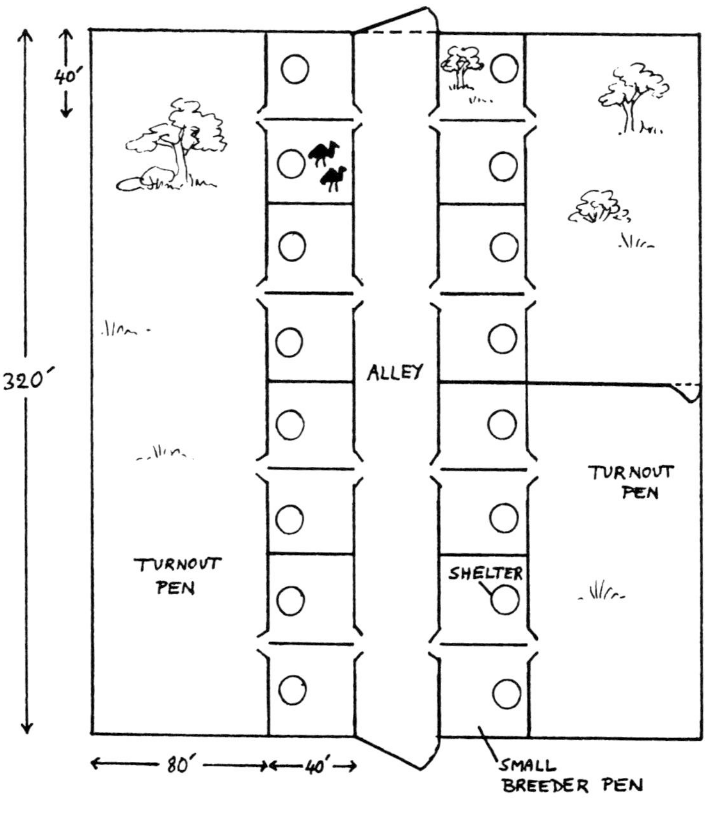

Fig. 2.1(b) - Smaller breeder pens with off-season pens.

disease a lot, due to the beneficial influences of sunshine and fresh air. However, being outside makes the birds more prone to irritation by insects, and insects can also spread disease. Insects multiply where droppings and/or muddy areas abound, so it is obviously in the farmer's best interests for the sake of insect control and animal health as well as for odor prevention, to keep standing water to a minimum. This can be done not only by good drainage but also by encouraging growth of vegetation.

A rotation system, whereby some pens are left empty for several months of the year to recover from trampling, can do wonders to ensure the continued health of animals in a farming operation. The pen system shown in **Fig. 2.1(b)** is ideal for this purpose. During breeding season, the birds are in small breeder pens and the larger area is left unused and in the off-season, the situation is reversed. Emu droppings provide excellent fertilizer, and whether pens are periodically reseeded or not, plants/grass will tend to grow which are deeper green and more lush, in areas where emus have been. Seeding pens with winter grass, such as rye grass, will provide a source of fresh greenery during the months when most other plants die due to frost. Even if this is not actually necessary in their diet, the grass again helps cope with emu droppings in the pen.

Additional suggestions/ideas

An important factor to consider in designing pens for breeders and chicks, is that if at all possible, chick pens should be separated from breeder pens. If this is not physically possible owing to lack of space, a visual barrier will need to be put up, whether in the form of a hedge, board fence, shade cloth or other barrier. A good idea might be to place breeder pens and chick pens on opposite sides of an existing barn or other building. There are many variations possible according to individual situations.

The reason for this separation is that the presence of young chicks can have several effects on the breeders:

1. Male becomes very possessive of chicks nearby, and loses interest in breeding the female.

2. Female stops laying eggs (whether because the male has lost interest, or due to the presence of chicks?)

3. Breeder birds may become more aggressive and start to fight, either with each other, or across the fence with other birds, or both.

4. Adult birds, in particular the male, becomes very stressed because he wants to be with the chicks. He may stop eating and become more nervous.

5. Adult birds may show aggression towards the chicks and pace the fence continually trying to get to them and chase them.

While none of this appears to have much of an effect on the chicks, (which probably recognize humans rather than adult emus as parent figures since they have been hand-raised) it can definitely be stressful to the breeding emus, and it would be better to avoid the situation completely. While the sound of chicks cheeping can stimulate some interest in the adult birds, the sight of them appears to have much more of an impact. Therefore, even if the chicks cannot be kept out of the sound range of the adults, keeping them out of sight should ensure that the adults are not unduly disturbed.

Once the breeding season is over, of course, this becomes much less important, and it does not matter if adults can see the older chicks/young birds in the growing-out pens.

Another factor to consider in breeder pen design is whether to use square pens or long narrow pens. We recommend that if pens are to be long, they should not be too narrow, or else in the course of walking the fence, all that will be left of the vegetation is a very thin strip. A square pen design not only ensures the growth of vegetation in the middle, but also provides more privacy to which the bird can retreat, away from humans or neighboring birds at the fence. For this reason, if long breeder pens are used, it would be advisable to make them at least 30' across.

The larger the size of the pen, the less its actual shape matters. The idea behind long narrow pens is to allow birds more running space (down the long sides of the pens) but in our experience, emus can run just as well in square pens since they look where they are going, negotiate turns easily and in general do not tend to run into fences unless chased and attempting to escape. Pens for young birds need to be larger all round than breeder pens, since the young birds need more exercise for proper bone and muscle growth and development.

2.4 IDENTIFICATION

Most emu farmers use legbands, or a combination of legbands and some permanent type of identification, to mark their birds. The permanent identification is either in the form of a microchip or a tattoo. While ostriches can be branded, this method would not work well on emus since they do not have bare skin on their thighs, but are feathered all over.

Permanent marking of birds helps to discourage theft as well as providing a means of identification, should a stolen or escaped bird be recovered. It is also useful in record-keeping, in order to compile breeding histories on birds (by keeping data on chicks) and for research purposes.

Marking of birds, in particular chicks and juveniles, will probably become less important as the commercial market develops and becomes established. At present, however, tagging and marking chicks enables follow-up to be done as regards later reproductive performance, performance on different feeds and many other factors which we need to learn more about.

(a) Tagging

Chicks can be tagged while still in the hatcher, to avoid confusion later if several are hatching on the same day. Since the first tag will need to be changed after a few weeks as the bird grows, an inexpensive home-made tag is usually the best choice. Numbered Velcro legbands or numbered plastic tags, held around the ankle with a cut-off cable tie, are methods commonly used. The biggest disadvantage to tagging chicks is the rate at which they grow. Tags must be replaced, or at least the tie holding the tag on, before they start to get too tight on the bird's leg and cause discomfort or any swelling.

Since ankle tags get stepped on a lot and are therefore more easily broken, tags can also be fastened just above the hock. Special care must be taken not to make it too tight (so it will cause no discomfort even when the bird is sitting) nor too loose, since it could slip down onto the actual hock and hamper the bird's movements. Any self-locking plastic band MUST have its trailing end cut off, so that there is no danger of it being pulled or stepped on which would tighten it further.

Wide plastic self-lock tags which are numbered and colored are often used for adult birds, again fastened either above the ankle or above the hock. Velcro tags are also used but become difficult to read with time, as dirt becomes ingrained and obscures the number. Plastic tags also eventually wear out and fall off, so they must be replaced periodically.

(b) Microchipping

The major advantage of microchipping is that it can be done at a very early age, and the bird never "grows out of" its microchip. The small possibility of irreparable damage to the chip by the bird crashing into something does exist, but can be offset by placing the chip in a less vulnerable location. Inserting the "chip" is much like giving an injection, and should be done by an experienced person. Microchipping may be done at hatching, or can be delayed until the bird's survival is certain, in order to save money. Microchips are not cheap and are not intended for re-use. A scanner is also needed in order to read microchip numbers. The scanner can be handheld, is usually battery-operated and scanning must be done fairly close to the bird in order to pick up the number. The main disadvantage of microchipping is its cost.

(c) Tattooing

A hand-held, battery operated pet tattooer which consists of a needle vibrating in and out of a "pen" at very high speed can be used for tattooing emus. The needle is dipped in ink at regular intervals and the numbers and/or letters are "written" on the bird's skin. The area under the wing is usually best, since there are fewer feathers there, and these can be plucked to provide adequate tattooing space. The process does not seem to cause much discomfort to the bird, although as always the bird will resist restraint from time to time. A good bird-handler is a necessity for successful tattooing. The tattooer is much cheaper than microchipping equipment, but is a lot more work. Also, it is best to wait until birds are at least 6 to 8 months old before tattooing, to allow for growth; so legbands will have to be relied on exclusively until then. However, tattooing unlike microchipping provides permanent marking that is also visible.

For marking (permanently) smaller numbers of birds, tattooing makes economic sense, whereas in larger operations where there are a lot more birds to be marked, the expense of microchipping equipment is probably justified, considering the amount of time and labor that will be saved.

2.5 EFFECTS OF OTHER LIVESTOCK

While it is not good farming practice to run several different species of animals in the same enclosure, no significant problems have been encountered with having other livestock (horses, sheep, cattle) in pens adjacent to emus. In such situations, however, the emus should be carefully watched for any signs of stress caused by the presence of the other animal(s).

Certain species of animal do seem to be viewed by emus as a threat and can have an inhibiting effect on breeding and egg production. Some farmers have reported this result when emus were kept in pens adjacent to ostriches, for example. The key factor in each situation would be to observe birds closely for any sign of stress, if it does become necessary to keep other animals close to the emu pens.

If the emu farmer also raises other species of birds, every effort should be made to keep the different types of birds separate from one another and enclosed. This will help to control the spread of any disease.

2.6 QUARANTINE

It is a good management practice to quarantine any new arrivals to the emu farm in pens that are separate from the breeder facilities for a period of at least 3 to 4 weeks. This gives the farmer a good opportunity to observe the new birds and get them acclimatized to their new situation as well as to ensure that they are healthy and will not carry any disease or problem to the rest of his flock. During this period birds can be wormed as a preventative measure, and any blood testing or other tests can be done. If there are no problems, the bird can be introduced to the regular facilities after this period.

CHAPTER 3

Handling and Moving Emus

3.1 HANDLING THE HEALTHY BIRD

Handling of emus is often necessary, so it is a good idea to become adept at it. Handling may be necessary for the following reasons:

- Moving birds (to new pens or into trailer for moving to new location)
- Sexing birds
- Medical treatment, when necessary
- Marking birds for identification purposes (e.g. tagging, tattooing or microchipping).

It is preferable to restrain the emu by holding it rather than attempting to put it in a chute or other restraining device, since the nature of the bird is to fight against restriction. A chute could pose a serious risk of injury to the bird.

With some practice, one person can usually handle an adult emu. Handling is something that must be done quickly and with the least fuss possible, so as not to upset the bird unnecessarily. Having birds that are fairly tame and used to human beings from the beginning is a great advantage, since such birds can usually be approached and caught fairly easily.

The most common way to handle adult-size birds is to approach the bird quietly (walk, do not run). Once you are close enough, grab it quickly and firmly from the side or behind by both wings. Allow the bird to get over its fright by letting it jump up and down a little while still keeping your hold on it. Then, if your purpose in catching the bird is to move it somewhere, propel it forward while moving behind or alongside it (still retaining your grip on its wings) so that the bird's energy is used for forward motion rather than jumping in attempts to escape.

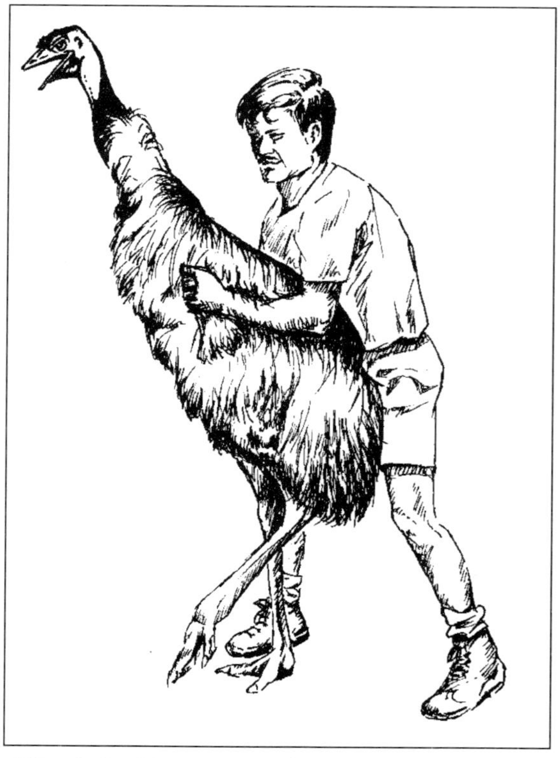

Fig. 3.1 - Moving an adult emu.

The best time of day to handle emus is early morning and late evening. Most birds will allow you to get close at these times, and more often than not you can quietly move them where you want them. Walk next to the bird to its destination, holding it as described, and if it is going up into a trailer, release the far side wing and, while still holding the near wing, boost it by its tailbone, propelling it firmly into the trailer filled with thick hay or straw. It is helpful to have an assistant ready to shut the gate at the instant the bird is in, so the bird does not have the opportunity to turn and attempt to jump out.

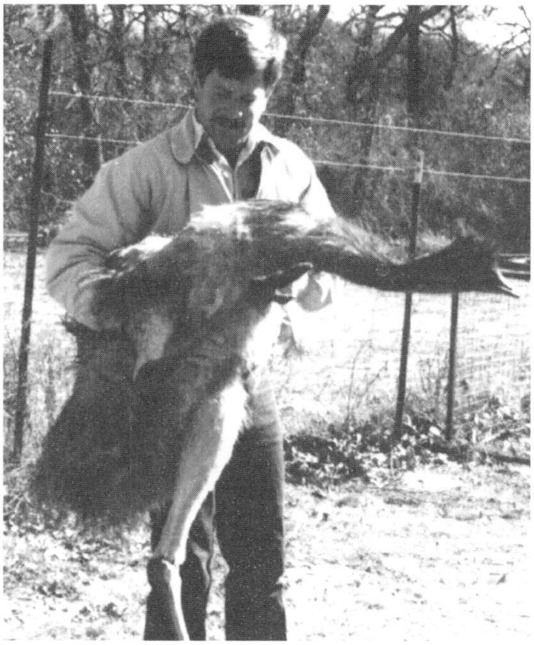

Plate 3.1 - Correct way to pick up and carry a bird.

Wild or nervous birds are sometimes a lot more difficult to deal with. To catch these type of birds in a pen, the best way is to corner the bird and give it a small gap to get by between you and the fence. As the bird goes by you, step forward and grab it in the usual way. It cannot get further away from you because of the fence. These birds will normally jump vigorously and kick, so be alert and stay with it, keeping your own legs out of the way to prevent being kicked. The worst birds like to back up under you, and if you maintain your grip on the wings, you may end up breaking them and/or the bird will end up on its back, kicking upwards at you. This is a quick way to be undressed and cut up by the flailing legs. The best way to deal with birds like these is to pick the bird up off the ground as soon as you lay hands on it. This is accomplished in the following way: Quickly slide one arm under the bird's leg, from behind, while the other arm slides across the front of the other leg. Clasp your hands across the bird's belly and immediately lift it, holding it firmly to your chest. After 4 to 6 kicks the bird usually ends up hanging limply in your grip. Carry it to the trailer and drop it forward onto its feet; quickly close the door.

It is better not to buy birds that are extremely wild and difficult to handle. While some do tame down, others never become quite as manageable as "normal" emus. Many wild birds also do not make good breeders as they do not settle down easily. If attempts to get the bird tame over a period of time fail, the owner of such a bird might consider fattening it for slaughter rather than continue to keep an unproductive bird that may also disrupt the peace of his other emus.

When the purpose of handling your emu is to hold it still (for sexing/treatment/marking) rather than to move it somewhere, catch it as described before and then attempt to keep it from jumping by leaning over its back, putting some (but not all) of your weight on it. Sometimes it helps to put slightly more weight on its one side than the other; that way the bird hopefully does not feel balanced enough to jump. Usually a tightening of its muscles will indicate that the bird wants to jump; slight release followed by continued pressure may help remind it that you are still holding it. Sometimes a blindfold (such as a dark sock or pillowcase over the bird's head) will help keep the bird quiet, but this does not always work. The person administering the treatment to the bird (e.g. tattooing, injecting etc.) should try to work as quickly and efficiently as possible, from the side and a little to the rear of the bird if possible in order to keep himself from getting kicked. He should also be prepared to jump out of the way in a hurry, should the handler have difficulty holding the bird still. Note that the most dangerous position to be in is usually directly in front of the bird, since its kick is forward. While jumping around, a backward swipe is also possible but is usually not as damaging. Note that emus seldom kick out of malice; they are simply trying to get away.

3.2 HANDLING THE SICK BIRD

Depending on the nature of its debilitation, the sick or injured emu may be either more or much less easy to handle than the normal, healthy bird. A very sick bird is usually quite docile, especially if he has been sick for a long time, as he will also be rather weak. Birds with injuries or stings to the eyes to the extent that vision is rather limited, will also tend to be docile and easily handled. However, once an eye that was gummed shut has been irrigated and treated to the extent that it can open and the bird can suddenly see, remember that he may get a great shock on seeing you, and may jump vigorously.

When a bird is injured and has lacerations that need to be stitched, he is often very wild and difficult to catch, as he is still keyed-up from the struggle with whatever it was that caused the injury. If an attempt is made at this point to tranquilize the bird with some form of injectable sedative, it may end up having the opposite effect, exciting him even more. This can be the case with other animals also (such as horses) and should be taken into consideration before making the decision to use a sedative.

RESTRAINT - If the sick bird cannot be "doctored" in a standing position, i.e. with one person holding the bird while the other administers medication, it may be restrained in a lying position, as follows:

1. While one person holds the bird, the other (wearing heavy gloves to prevent his hands from being "rasped" by the bird's scaly legs) grasps the bird's legs, about halfway between hock and ankle, and holds them together. Note: a firm grip is needed (use both hands) as the bird may struggle at this point.

2. The bird-holder and the leg-holder together gently lower the bird to the ground, on its side.

3. The leg-holder keeps the bird's legs together and bent towards its belly, exerting some pressure in that direction to prevent the bird kicking out, while the bird-holder (or other person) may now administer medication. The bird's legs may be lifted slightly, so that the bird is lying partly on its back, partly on its side. This is sometimes an easier position from which to exert pressure.

4. When finished with the bird, the leg-holder swings the bird's legs over to roll

the bird onto its belly; then he gets out of the way quickly in case the bird flails its legs before getting up.

If a person has to restrain a bird alone in an emergency situation, a wide nylon strap or strong belt may be used to hold the bird's legs together. After the bird has been pulled down on its side, the strap is passed across the bird's back and held from the other side. This keeps the legs tucked up against it. If the bird manages to get its legs underneath it, it may be able to stand up, so make sure both legs stay on one side.

If a bird needs to be tube-fed, the standing position is best, to make sure that nothing goes into the windpipe by mistake. Superficial wounds that require stitching may be done in the lying position, using local anesthetic. Sexing can be done either way, depending on the experience of the handler. If he can determine sex by feel only and does not need to see the organs, he can usually accomplish the procedure with the bird standing.

A bird suspected to be egg-bound should be handled with more care than usual, so as to minimize the slight but nevertheless possible risk of breaking the egg inside her and thus causing damage to her oviduct.

3.3 HANDLING CHICKS AND JUVENILES

Very young chicks can be easily held and carried with two hands, one on either side of the body, with legs tucked up or dangling between fingers. They can also be scooped up from the front, hand under chest and belly, the other hand steadying the chick over the back. Sometimes if a chick is struggling, tilting the neck and head downwards helps to quieten it. Groups of young chicks may be carried in a cardboard box, hamper or pet carrier - keeping in mind to keep the top of any container covered, as the chicks will do their utmost to jump out. A non-slip floor such as hay, straw, towels or rubber matting should always be provided to prevent any leg injuries due to slipping.

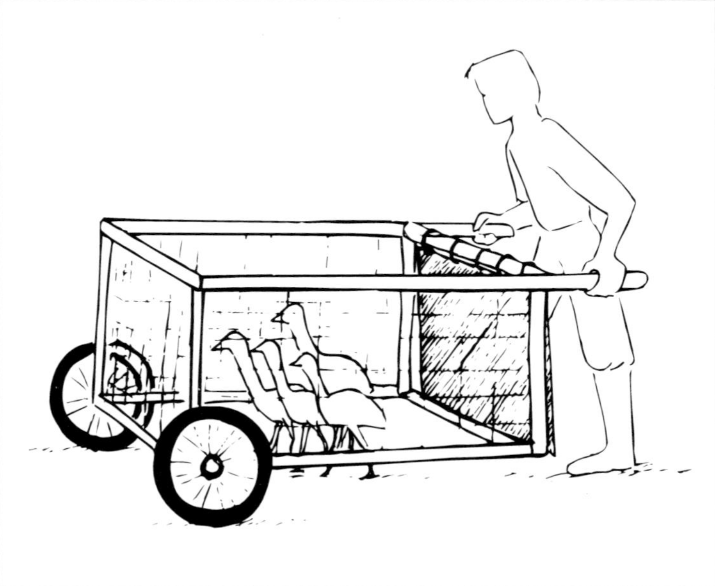

Fig. 3.2 - Example of a "walking cage" for moving young birds. A person walking in front with a feed bucket is helpful.

From about two months old, chicks will have grown enough to be difficult to carry in the hands; also, their flailing toenails can give the handler a couple of good scratches. The easiest and safest way to carry the bird at this point (both for the bird and for the handler) is by catching the bird, grasping both legs (while it is standing) firmly about half-way between hock joint and ankle joint and, making sure to hold the legs together, lift the bird so that it hangs upside-down, while supporting it at the base of the neck. Should the bird be able to get one leg free, not only may the bird get injured but the handler also is bound to collect a few scratches on his hand/arm as the loose leg flails. To put the bird down, lay it on its side, wait for it to quieten down and stop struggling, then release your grip and step back, allowing the bird to get to its feet on its own.

3.4 HANDLING YOUNG BIRDS

Young birds from 6 to 18 months old are probably the most difficult of all to handle. They tend to be much more feisty than a settled, mature emu, and are of course much more of a handful than a smaller chick. Several instances have occurred where, in kicking and flailing while at the same time lowering its head to try to get away or because it is being picked up, a bird has managed to tear a gash in its own neck. This may damage the esophagus, the windpipe, or both. If it occurs, a veterinarian is usually needed to sew the bird up. Since prevention is of course better than cure, the main thing to think about when moving young birds is not to let the neck get in the way of the legs, and to move the birds by running them rather than by lifting and carrying them. If it is necessary to hold the bird (e.g. for sexing) rather than move it, have an assistant hold or strap the legs together near the ankles so that the bird cannot kick. The bird may be restrained in this way either standing or gently laid on its side.

3.5 THE ESCAPEE

There are few emu farmers who have never had a bird get out of where it was supposed to be - whether it escaped from a pen, a trailer or as a result of a gate being left open. An escaped bird will often head for heavy brush where, unfortunately, it is able to move a lot faster than human beings. An aid in catching such a bird, if moving fairly slowly, is to arouse its curiosity - squat or crouch down (to present less of a threat to the bird), move something around on the ground with your hand (e.g. a shiny or brightly colored object), or pour some corn chops (highly visible and attractive to emus) on the ground while the emu is looking at you, if you happen to have some with you. If you cannot get close enough to grab him in this way, you may have to follow the bird till he reaches a fence-line, which he will probably start to walk along, according to emu custom. You should then be able to catch him against the fence in the usual way. (If the bird is used to the sight of a feed bucket, you may be able to get him to follow you with feed.)

Many people who have never handled emus before are more than willing to assist in catching an escaped bird. It is important to instruct them in how to catch and hold the bird before embarking on the chase, both for their own safety and that of the emu. An emu can sustain severe internal injuries if tackled and thrown to the ground, football-fashion, by a well-meaning but over-enthusiastic "helper".

3.6 HERDING EMUS

Although emus tend to move in a group when in larger numbers, they are notoriously difficult to actually herd or "drive". The reason is that the emu's reaction on feeling himself pushed or driven anywhere, is usually to turn and try to crowd past the person(s) attempting to drive him forward. In this way a flock usually scatters, running towards and past their pursuers (or in any direction except where you want them to go), rather than bunching together like cattle or sheep and moving away from the pressure.

Moving a large number of emus by foot to a new area is best accomplished by the use of alleys or runways. If not already in place, temporary runways can be made using sturdy cattle panels or similar materials. The group of emus will be most easily moved if they can be encouraged to move of their own volition. A highly visible feed, such as cracked corn (corn chops) can be of great help; small piles of it can be poured at regular intervals along the alley. If the emus will follow a person walking ahead with a feed bucket, so much the better. A second person is necessary to bring up the rear, to prevent the emus from going back again. The person in the rear may carry a panel the width of the alley to keep it closed off behind the emus, or may carry two poles to wave above his head and thus, hopefully, deter any emus who want to turn back and crowd past him. Watching an emu for signs of what he is going to do is important here. If you run towards an emu who is already moving in your direction, chances are he will increase his efforts to crowd past you. If you stop, raise your arms and then stand still, he will often hesitate too. Once he has stopped, it is possible to get him to turn around and move away from you - e.g. by waving your arms slightly, jumping a little on the spot, or making a noise. However, as soon as you "crowd" him (get too close) he will try to get past you. That "safe distance" at which he will move away from you rather than towards you is something that can only be learned by keen observation and experience, but it usually does not take long to figure out. Of course, if several birds decide to run in your direction at once, you have lost your edge and will probably have to start over; you can intimidate a single bird but usually not a group.

3.7 HELPFUL HAULING HINTS

Emus can be hauled in stock trailers or utility trailers, and tend to be least stressed if hauled by night. The darkness usually helps in getting them to settle down quickly and simply go to sleep. In the heat of summer, hauling in the evening hours is especially helpful, since the air is cooler and there is usually little danger of heat stress. Hauling at mid-day in the baking heat is never a good idea with any animal, and if you have to do so, it may be advisable to stop at regular intervals to give the birds fresh water and, if they are stressed and panting heavily to hose them down. Watch for signs of trampling, such as one bird staying down (due to injuries/stress) when all others get up.

To haul emus with the greatest amount of safety and comfort, the trailer (or container, in the case of chicks) should be:

- Fairly dark - darkness helps settle birds down. A closed-in trailer is always vastly preferable to an open stock trailer.

- Well ventilated, but not to the extent that the birds are hit by the full force of the wind. (Again, most closed-in trailers fit the requirements, whereas open trailers do not.)

- Free of protuberances upon which the birds can injure themselves, or slats between which a leg or neck could slip and break.

- Well padded with a non-slip surface such as a thick layer of straw or hay. Well-fed emus do not usually attempt to eat their bedding materials, so there is little risk of intestinal impaction.

- Compartmented, if a large group of emus are being hauled, to reduce risk of birds piling on top of one another, causing suffocation/injury.

- Easily and properly latched. Easy opening and closure is a great aid in loading and unloading the birds. The latch must also be safe, so there is no risk of any doors flying open during travel. Finally, if a person has to stop anywhere for the night, a chain and lock to further secure his valuable cargo might also be a wise idea.

One additional factor to consider if hauling young chicks, is of course warmth. Chicks are more susceptible to chilling than are adult birds, which already have a protective layer of fat covering their bodies in addition to a thick layer of feathers. Therefore, make sure the chicks are not in a draught or shivering. Thick hay, a good sturdy container or box, and a few fellow chicks with whom to share body heat will help keep chicks comfortable when being transported, whether by road or by air freight.

If hauling by night and the journey takes no longer than one night, it is usually not necessary to stop in order to feed/water the emus. On longer journeys, however, this will be necessary, and one should be prepared for this by bringing the proper feed and containers. While some adult emus may not want to eat on the journey, they will probably want water at some point on a long trip. Adding poultry vitamins/electrolytes to the water may help alleviate effects of stress, provided the birds will drink it.

CHAPTER 4

Anatomy of the Emu

*The study of an animal's anatomy can be a key to understanding more about the animal itself. For example, the structure of an animal's digestive system will usually give a very good indication of what sort of dietary requirements it has, as will be seen later (**Section 6.1 - 6.3**). In addition, although every emu farmer cannot be an animal doctor, he/she will almost certainly have to become a fairly competent animal nurse at some point. Therefore, a basic knowledge of the structure and functions of the animal's body is essential.*

4.1 THE SKELETON

The skeleton of the emu is the framework on which its body is built. It provides strength and support for the muscles attached to it, and protection for the brain, spinal cord and other sensitive organs which it encases.

Fig. 4.1 shows the skeleton of a 3-month-old emu. In the adult, it is possible that some of the parts labelled as "cartilage" might later ossify (harden into bone). The bones of a fully grown adult would also be somewhat thicker; other than that, there should not be much difference in skeletal structure. The parts are as follows:

SKULL

1. Lower mandible
2. Upper mandible (beak)
3. External naris (nostril)
4. Orbit (eye socket)
5. Brain case

NECK

6. Cervical (neck) vertebrae - there were 18 on this specimen including the small, ring-shaped ATLAS which articulates with the skull.

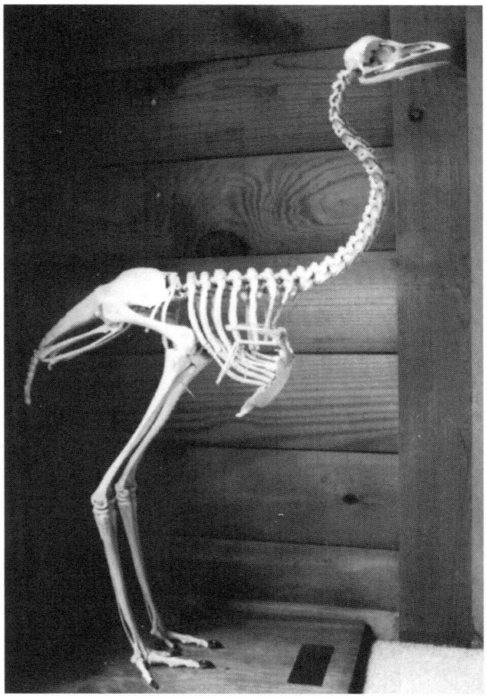

Plate 4.1 - Skeleton of 3 to 4 month emu.

Fig. 4.1 - Skeleton of the emu.
(3 months old)

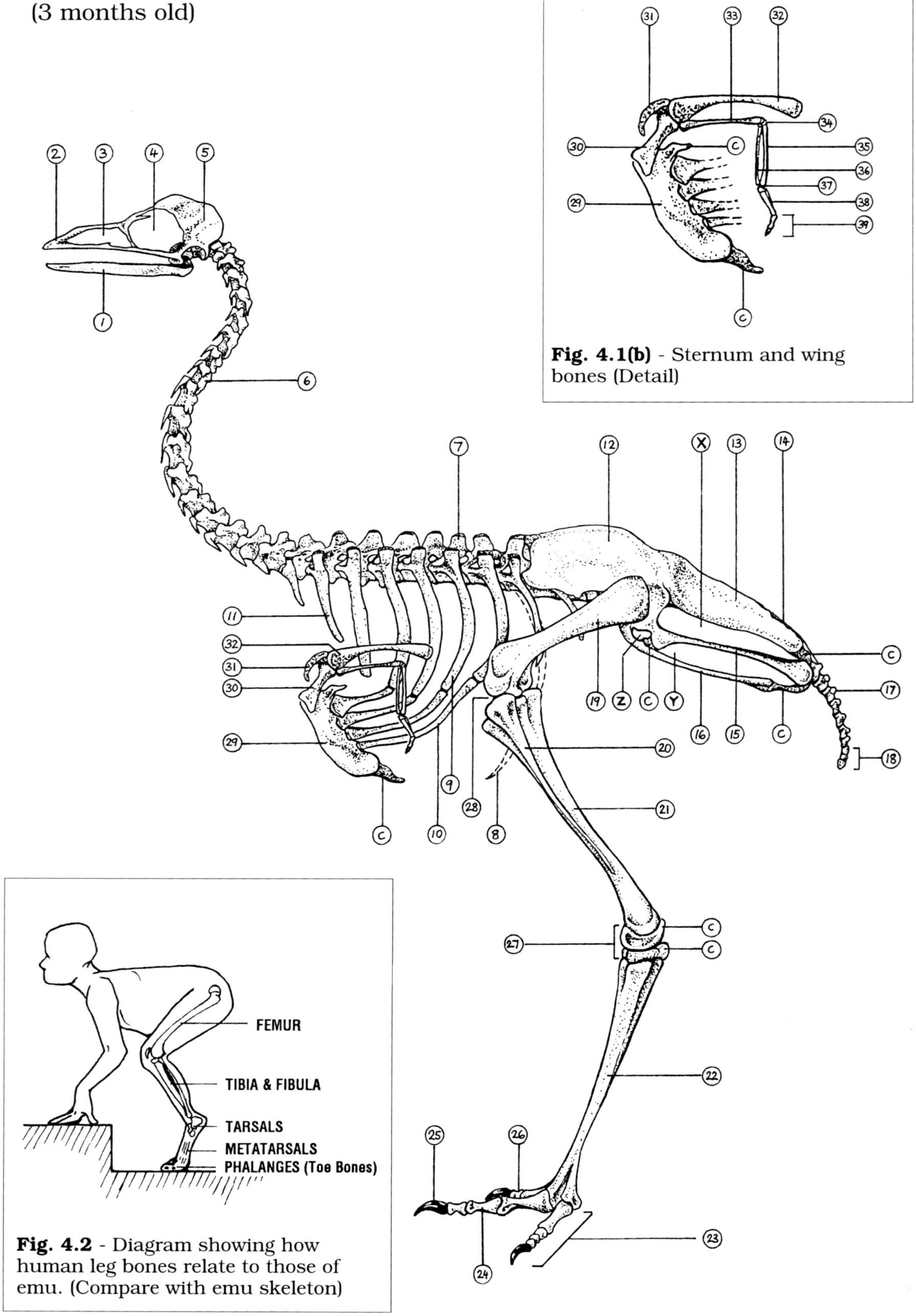

Fig. 4.1(b) - Sternum and wing bones (Detail)

Fig. 4.2 - Diagram showing how human leg bones relate to those of emu. (Compare with emu skeleton)

THORAX AND ABDOMEN

7. Thoracic vertebra. (These vertebrae articulate with the ribs)

8. Long floating 8th rib on right side made up of 2 components in the usual way, but lower component does not appear to attach to sternum. Left corresponding rib much shorter and only has vertebral component. Interesting feature, perhaps sex-related? (This specimen's sex was unknown.)

9. Rib - vertebral component

10. Rib - sternal component

11. Floating rib, i.e. has no sternal component

PELVIS

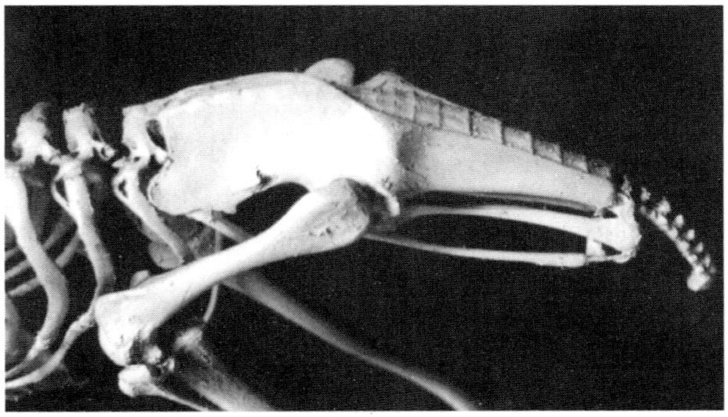

Plate 4.2 - Top view of the synsacrum.

12. Ilium (preacetabular, meaning in front of the acetabulum, which is the cup-shaped socket into which the head of the femur fits).

13. Ilium (postacetabular, i.e. behind the acetabulum)

14. Synsacrum, caudal part. (The synsacrum begins under the ilium, is fused to it and consists of fused thoracic, lumbar, sacral and caudal vertebrae).

15. Ischium

16. Pubis

TAIL

17. Caudal vertebrae

18. Pygostyle (end tailbone, consisting of several fused caudal vertebrae)

LEG

19. Femur - articulates with pelvis at hip joint. This joint permits rotation as well as protraction, retraction, abduction and adduction.

20. Fibula

21. Tibiotarsus (also known as tibia)

22. Tarsometatarsus (also known as metatarsus)

The fact that in addition, different textbooks may call either of these bones "tarsus" can be rather confusing.

23. Digit (outer toe) consisiting of 5 phalanges. The phalanges are the small bones of each toe. Note that the toenails are also phalanges, somewhat modified.

24. Phalanx of middle toe. This toe has a total of 4 phalanges.

25. Toenail (a modified phalanx) of middle toe.

26. Phalanx of 3rd digit (inner toe). This toe has only 3 phalanges.

27. Hock (tarsal joint). Flexion and extension takes place in this joint.

28. Knee joint, capable of flexion and extension. A small, triangular patella ("kneecap" - not shown) lies embedded in the thick cartilage at the front of this joint.

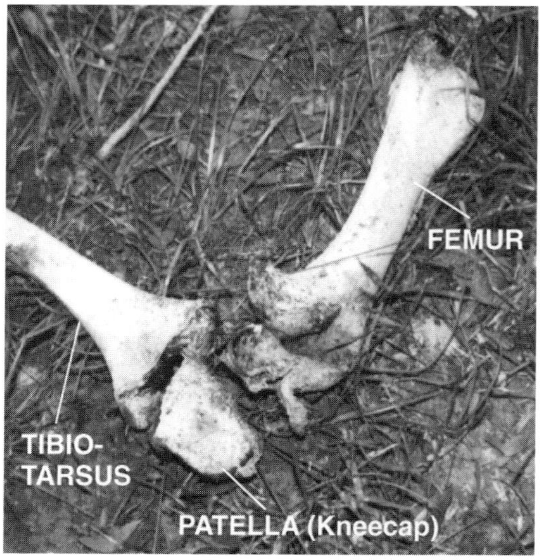

Plate 4.3 - Position of Patella (kneecap) - adult emu.

STERNUM AND WING

(This key corresponds both with whole skeleton drawing and with inset **Fig. 4.1(b)**. Inset shows wing bones in greater detail.)

29. Sternum (breastbone)

30. Coracoid

31. Clavicle

32. Scapula (shoulderblade) - attached firmly to rib cage by thin layer of muscle

33. Humerus

34. Elbow joint

35. Ulna. In most birds, the ulna is thicker than the radius.

36. Radius

37. Carpal joint

38. Carpometacarpus

39. Single digit, with 2 phalanges

FORAMENS

A foramen, or fenestra, is simply an opening in the bone. These openings are useful in allowing nerves, tendons etc. to pass through.

X Ilioschiadic foramen

Y Ischiopubic fenestra

Z Obdurator foramen

C - indicates CARTILAGE, some of which may later ossify into bone when the bird matures into an adult.

The Spinal Column

The spinal column can be divided up as follows:

1. CERVICAL vertebrae - 18, including the ring-shaped atlas which articulates with the skull. (Chickens generally have 16 neck vertebrae; swans may have 20 or more.) This large number of neck vertebrae (compared with only 7 in mammals) allows for great flexibility in the bird's neck, allowing it to pick up food in its beak with accuracy and ease. The neck is S-shaped, as in most birds.

2. THORACIC vertebrae - 8 free thoracic vertebrae, as well as 2 which form part of the synsacrum and are under the ilium.

3. SYNSACRUM - consists of fused vertebrae, as follows: Thoracic - 2; Lumbar - 12; Sacral - 4; Caudal - 2; giving a total of 20 fused vertebrae (in this specimen).

4. CAUDAL vertebrae - 7 free caudal vertebrae, followed by 2 or 3 fused caudal vertebrae which form the end tailbone (known as "pygostyle" in poultry.) The free caudal vertebrae allow movement of the tail, as in raising the tail for preening or mating.

Note that these numbers have all been based on one specimen, and in birds some variations in the number of vertebrae (especially the neck) may occur. Nevertheless, this specimen should give a good representation of its species. For instance, the fact that the thoracic vertebrae are free and not fused (as in the chicken) explains how it is possible for an emu to develop a deformed spine which curves sideways. It is likely that any nutritional deficiency which causes a curved neck in the chicken, would cause a curved neck and spine in the emu, since it is possible for its spine to curve.

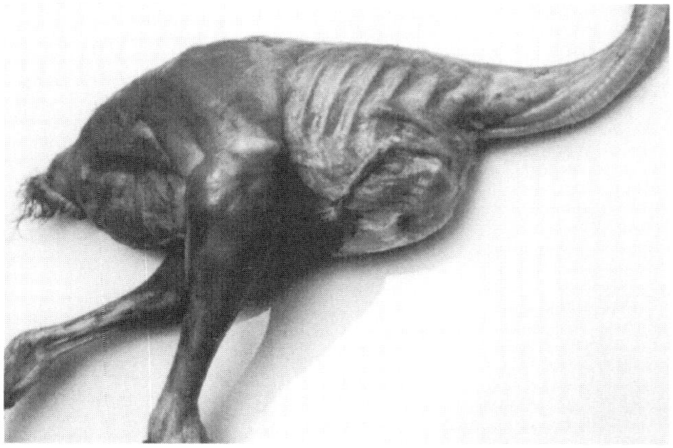

Plate 4.4 - Top layer of muscles (directly under the skin) of 3-month-old emu.

4.2 MUSCLES

The study and identification of the muscles of the emu is fertile ground for further research. (**Plate 4.4**) shows the arrangement of the external muscles (just under the skin), in particular of the leg.

4.3 STRUCTURAL DIFFERENCES BETWEEN EMU (A RATITE) AND FLYING BIRDS (CARINATES)

It is interesting to note some of the differences between the skeleton of the emu and that of a flying bird, such as the chicken or pigeon. As one might expect, the structural differences have a lot to do with the flight capabilities (or lack thereof) of the bird. Here are some examples:

1. **Sternum (breastbone)** - In the chicken, this bone has a deep "keel" for the attachment of the strong flight muscles (the white meat on a chicken-breast). The emu's sternum has no such keel but is rounded and smooth like a shallow bowl. There is no breast meat on an emu because there are no flight muscles. The same is true of the ostrich and rhea. The word "ratite" which is used to describe this family of large, non-flying birds comes from the Latin word "ratis", meaning "raft". It is a description of this flat breastbone, comparing it with that of "carinate" birds whose sternum has a keel like a boat (from the Latin "carina" meaning "keel".)

2. **Ribs** - Flying birds often have ribs with a second "branch", or "uncinate process" which overlaps onto the next rib and helps give strength and rigidity to the skeleton for the stresses experienced while flying. The emu's ribs have no such processes but are more like the ribs of a land mammal.

3. **Thoracic vertebrae** - Most of the chicken's thoracic vertebrae are fused, again to lend further strength and rigidity to the skeleton for flight. The emu's thoracic vertebrae are not fused, not only because it does not fly but also probably because the added flexibility of the back is a better adaptation for running.

4. **Wings** - Of course, the wings themselves in the emu are very much reduced both in size and number of digits compared with other birds, since they serve no useful purpose.

5. **Clavicles** - Again, these bones and any muscles surrounding them are very much reduced in the emu. In the chicken, the clavicles are fused in front to form the "wishbone" (furcula), and the muscles attached to it provide additional support for flying. In this emu specimen, only a thin band of cartilage joined the two separated clavicles in front.

6. **Leg bones** - The emu's leg bones are well adapted to running, with a short thick femur and long, strong tibiotarsus and tarsometatarsus.

7. **Toes** - Reduction in the number of toes is also an adaptation for running. All the toes face forward as the emu does not perch, and therefore has no need of a supporting toe or toes facing backwards.

8. **Overall structure** - The emu's body is well balanced, long rather than deep, and well streamlined for ease in running.

9. **Pneumatic bones** - While the bones of flying birds are often "pneumatized" (have air spaces in them to reduce overall body weight - another adaptation for flight) it is possible that the bones of the emu are not pneumatized to the same degree. Not enough research has been done yet on this matter, but it could be of importance in the treatment of air sacculitis, since harmful organisms which invade the air sacs of a bird also sometimes invade the air spaces in the bones. It would be interesting to find out to what extent this could occur in the emu.

4.4 THE DIGESTIVE TRACT

Fig. 4.3 is a representation of the digestive tract of the emu. The relative size and positioning of various parts of the gut is as close as possible to the bird in real life; however, for the sake of clarity, the length of intestine between gizzard and anus has been shortened in this diagram. In an actual specimen there are many more loops and coils, but they occupy approximately the same space.

The membrane that envelops the whole gut system and holds it together is called the PERITONEUM. There are also membranes between various loops of the intestine that hold them together and supply the intestine with a rich network of blood vessels for uptake of nutrients from the gut. The blood then transports these nutrients to the rest of the body as needed. Blood vessels and membranes are not shown in the diagram but can be seen in **Plate 4.5**.

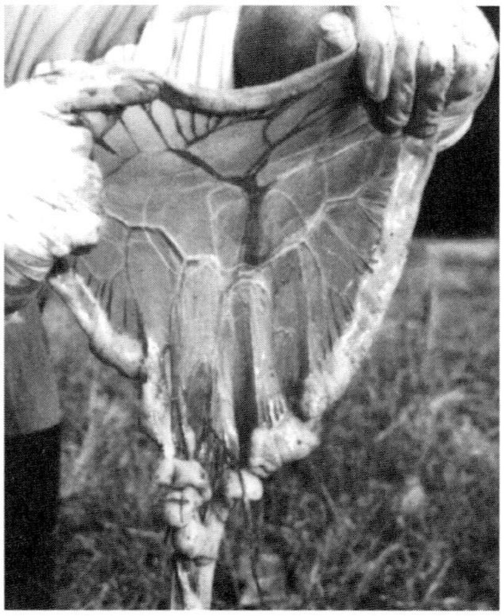

Plate 4.5 - Membranes with network of blood vessels surrounding intestines.

Parts of the digestive tract.

1. Esophagus (gullet)
2. Proventriculus
3. Ventriculus (gizzard)
4. Duodenum, first section, U-shaped
5. Jejunum
6. Diverticulum (remnant of the yolk sac)
7. Ileum

(4–7: SMALL INTESTINE)

8. Juncture of small intestine with large intestine
9. Paired ceca
10. Colon (referred to as "rectum" in some texts)

(9–10: LARGE INTESTINE)

11. Cloaca

12. Anus (vent)

A - Opening of trachea (windpipe), in bottom of mouth.

B - Place where trachea divides into two bronchi and the esophagus passes between these two bronchi.

C - Pancreas.

Functions of various parts of the digestive system.

1. **Esophagus** - This is a tube with very elastic walls through which food and water are passed, after being swallowed, to the rest of the gut for digestion. The inner surface of the esophagus has many longitudinal folds, which also helps increase the inner surface area and elasticity, so that large particles can be swallowed without lodging in the throat or causing harm to the bird.

Lubrications secreted into the esophagus also help food to pass down more easily. Note that the emu has no crop. In birds that have crops, this is a sac-like structure in the front of the neck which is part of the esophagus. Its main purpose is the storage and softening of food, either for later use by the bird or for regurgitation to feed helpless young or court a mate. The emu does not regurgitate as part of its courting behavior, nor does it need to feed its young, since the chicks are hatched able to pick up food by themselves. Note: It is important to know the position of the esophagus in case the bird is ill enough to need tube-feeding. If food/water are mistakenly tubed into the TRACHEA instead of the esophagus, the bird will usually die. (see **Section 14.10** for proper method of tube-feeding).

2. **Proventriculus** - The glandular stomach, where enzymes are secreted onto the food and digestion begins. The proventriculus looks mottled on the outside, giving a "textured" appearance similar to the kidneys, but is lighter in color than the kidneys. It is a creamy-beige to pinkish color. The walls in cross-section consist of many tubules, packed together like a bunch of spaghetti cut into short lengths.

3. **Gizzard, or Ventriculus** - A large, rounded structure which is very muscular and thick-walled and usually feels hard to the touch, especially if the bird has recently eaten. This organ serves as the bird's "teeth" since it grinds up food into smaller, more digestible particles. The grinding action is accomplished by the combined action of the muscular gizzard walls and small stones or bits of gravel that have been ingested. Therefore, if a bird does not have access to stones or some such type of grit, its ability to grind up food will be severely reduced, and IMPACTION may result (see **Section 14.5(a)**). The gizzard in cross-section resembles the cross-section of a fig. Its inner sac follows the contours of the outer, muscular portion but is a separate entity which can be easily peeled away from the outer muscular layer on dissection. The inner sac appears continuous with the intestine, and has many folds on its inside. It is usually stained a

Fig. 4.3 - Digestive System of emu (3 months old).

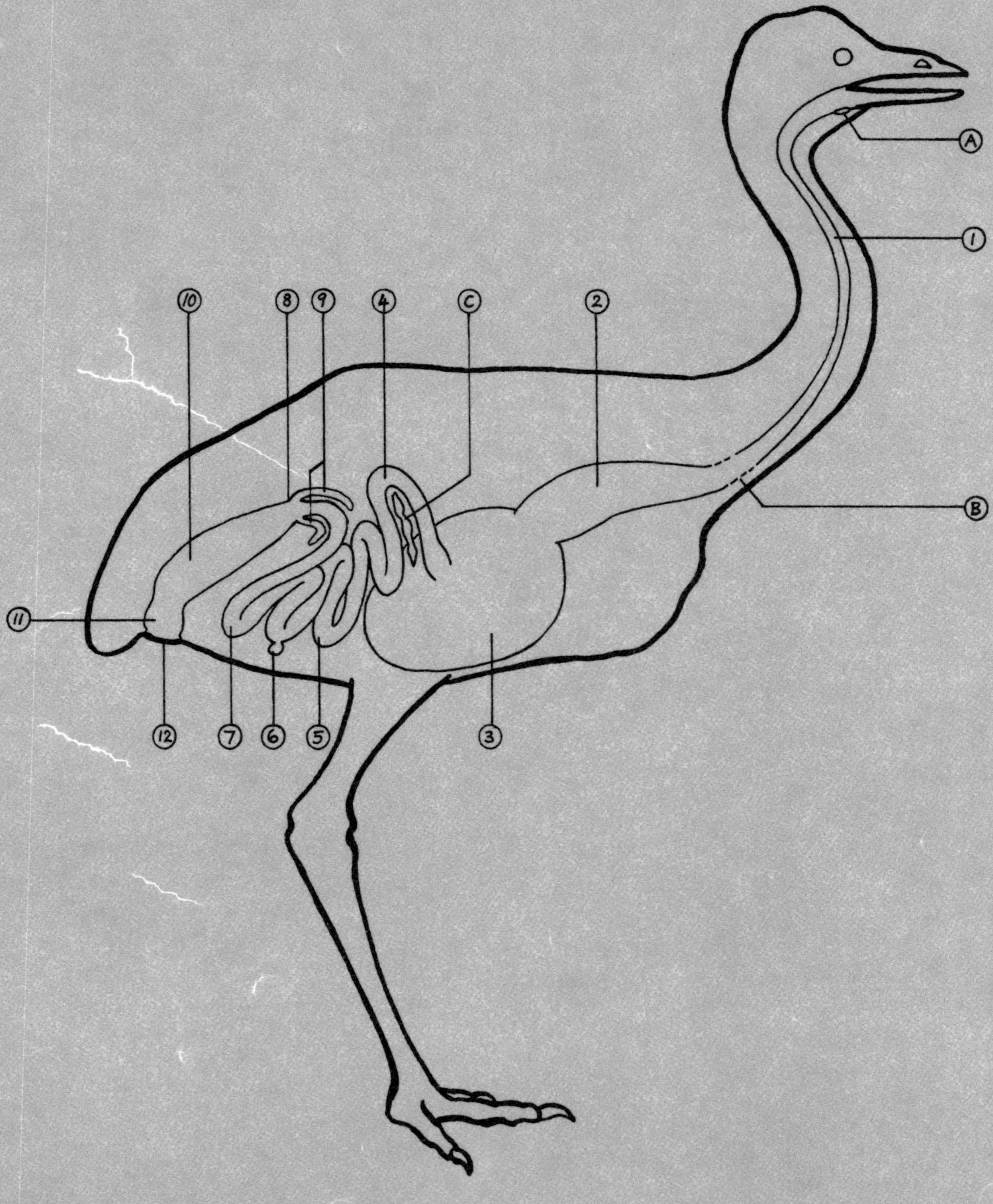

Fig. 4.3 - Digestive System of emu (3 months old).

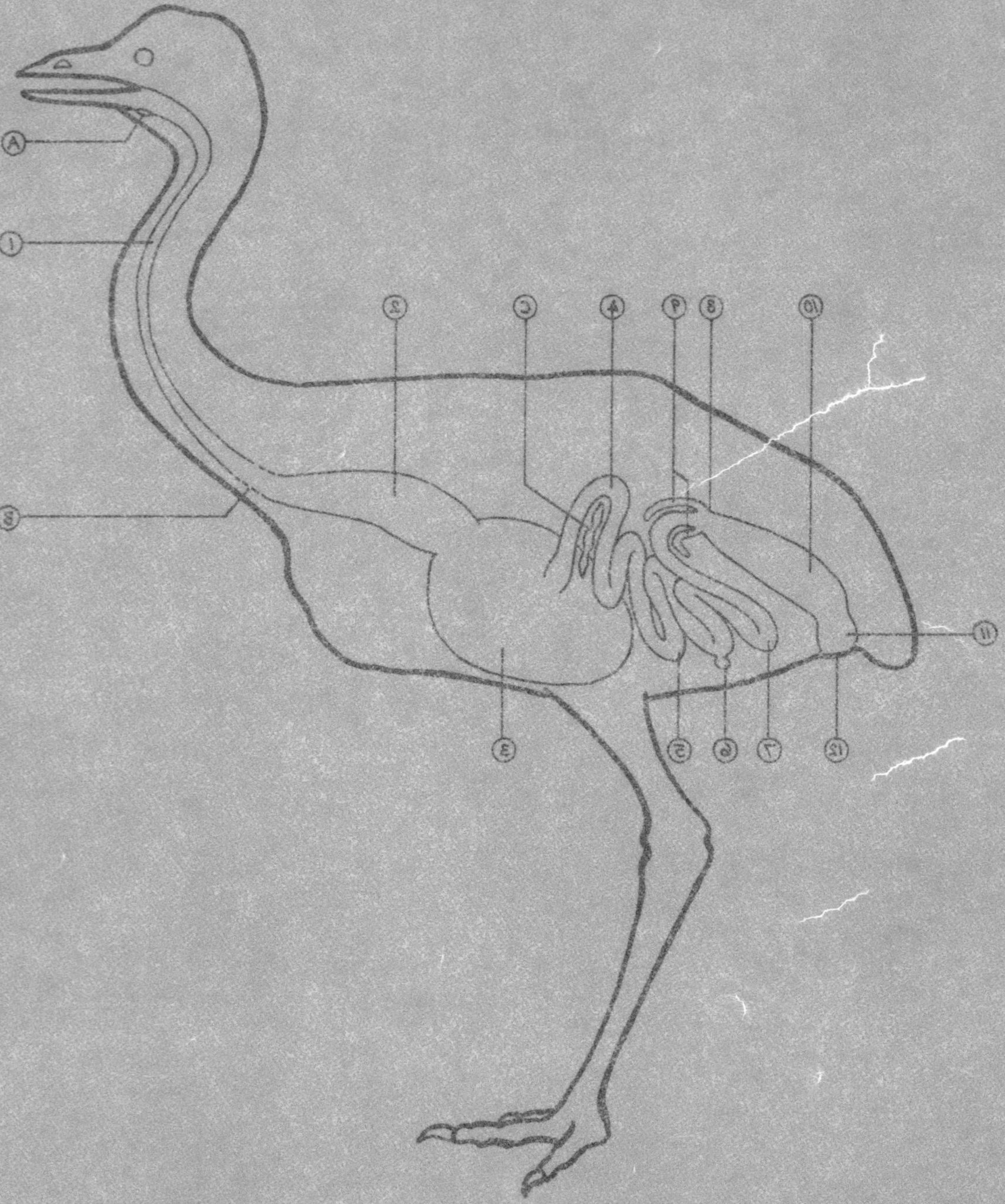

Fig. 4.4 - Major organs of emu (3 months old).

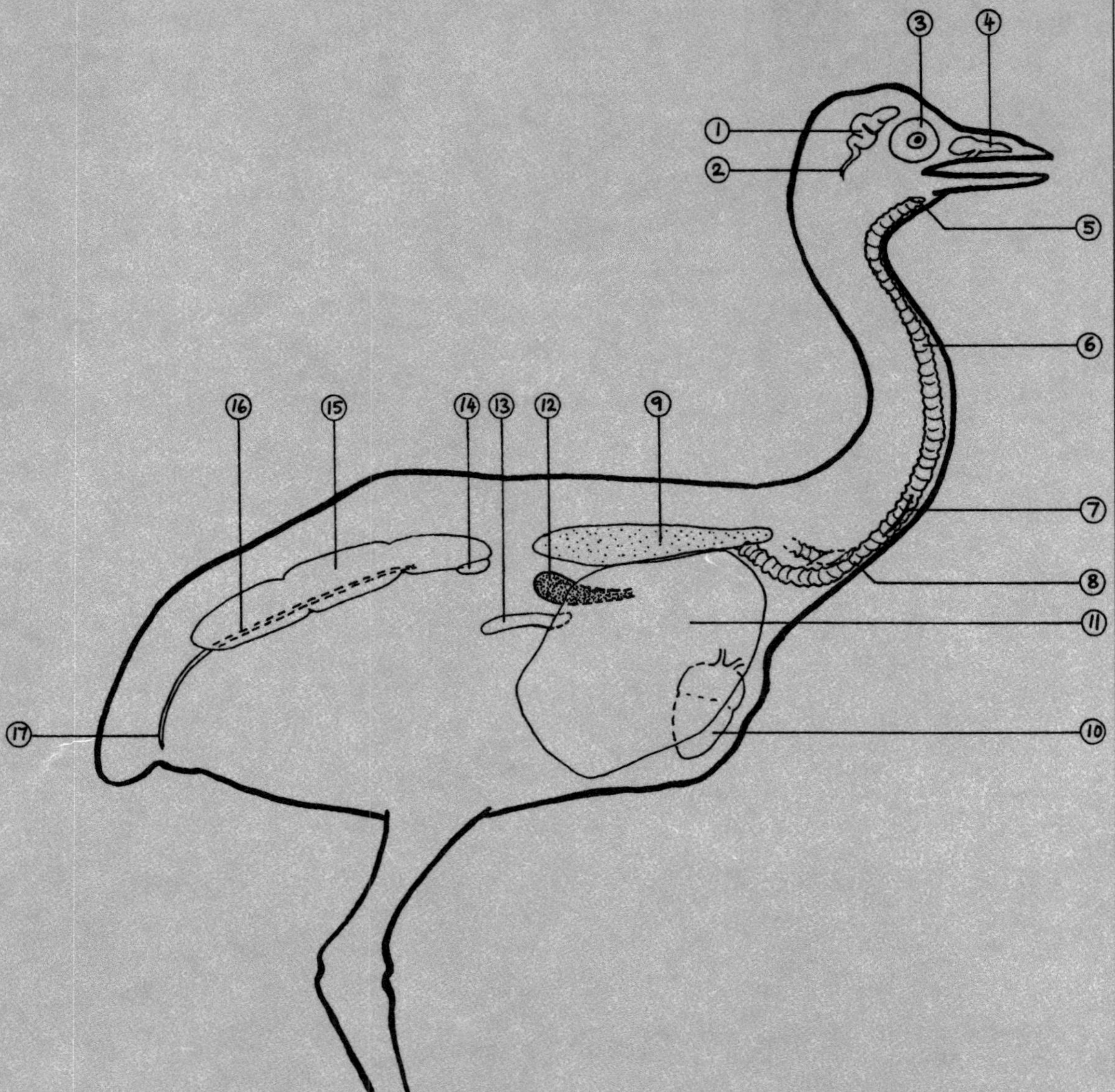

Fig. 4.4 - Major organs of emu (3 months old).

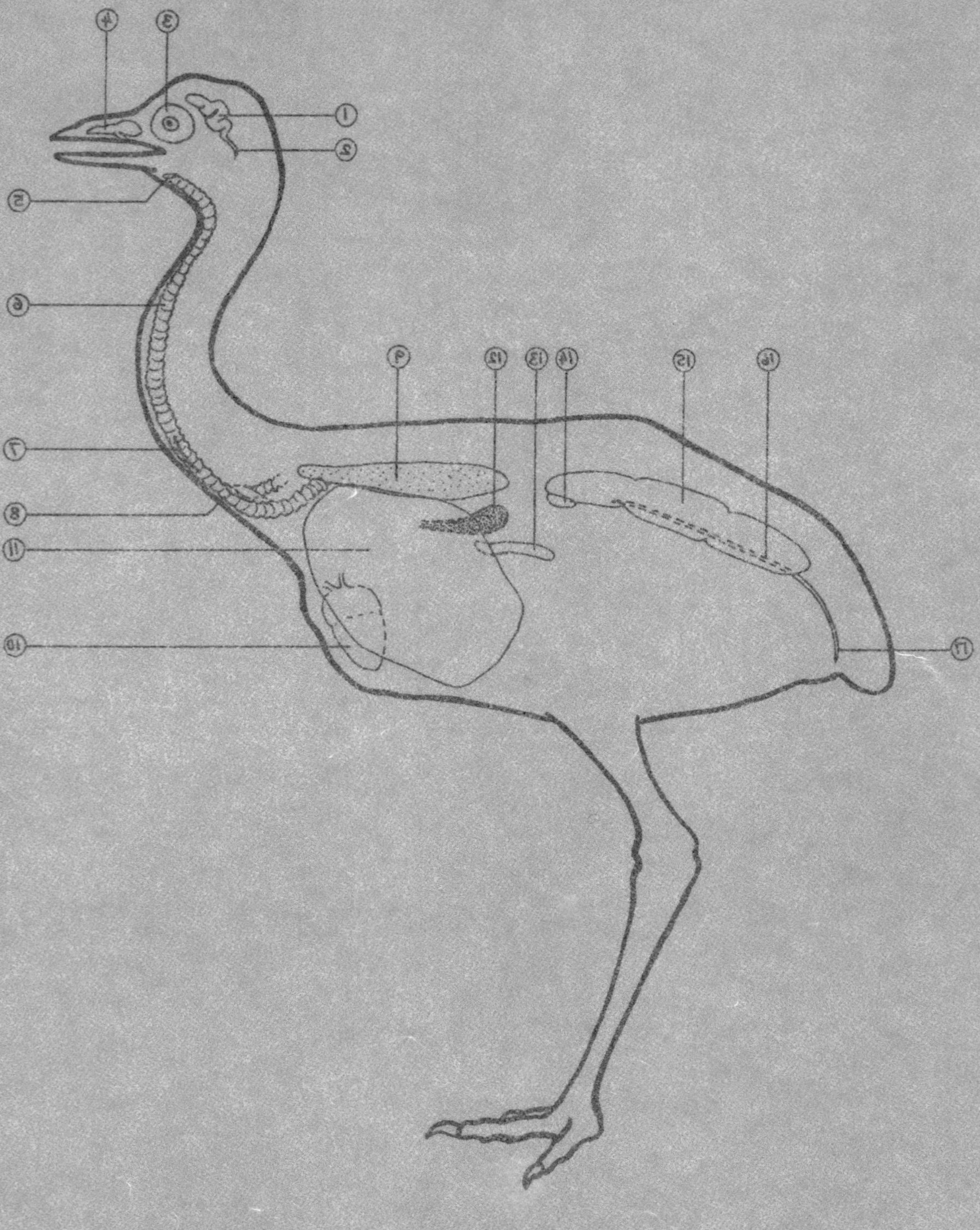

Fig. 4.1 - Skeleton of the emu. (3 months old).

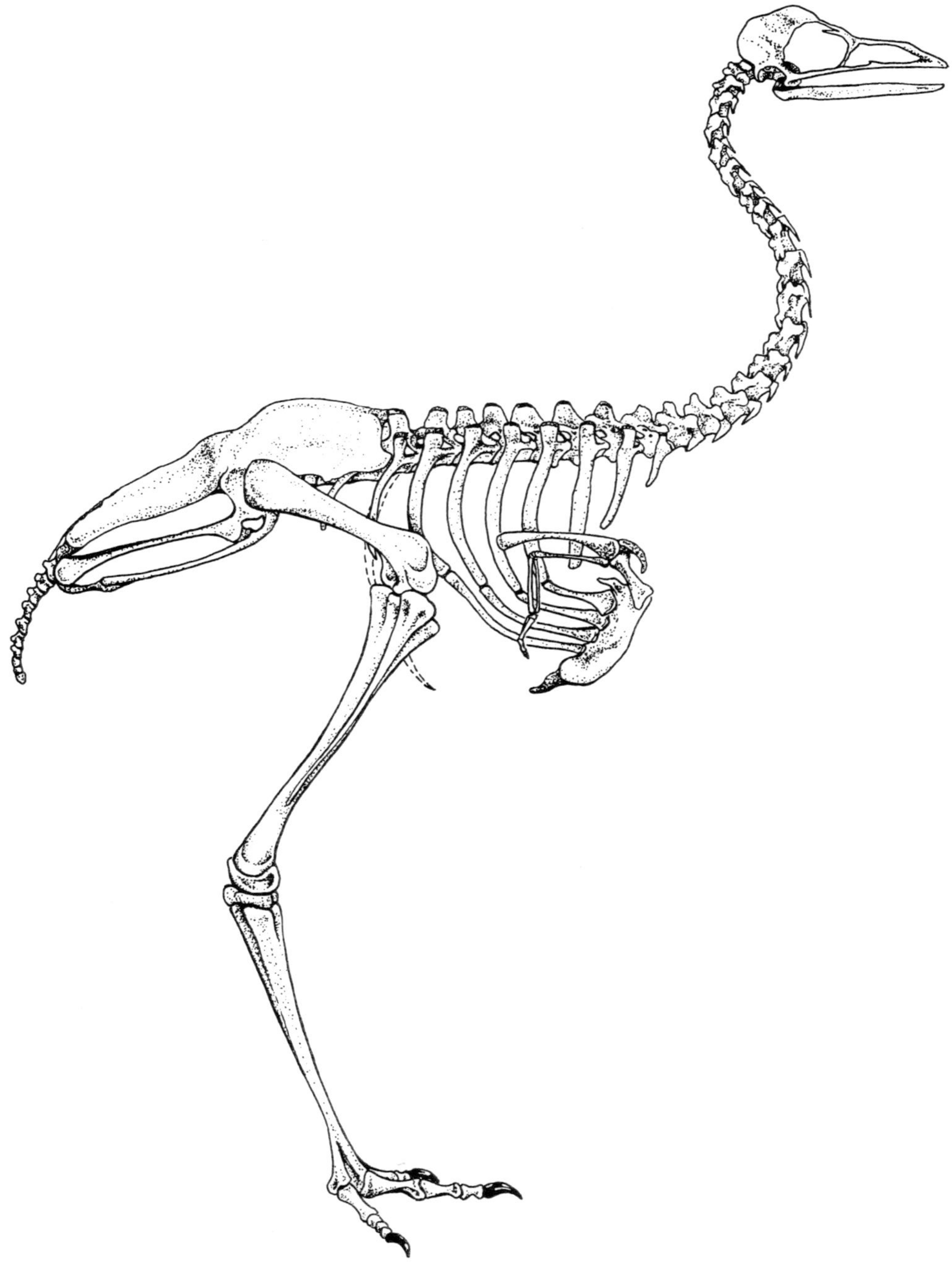

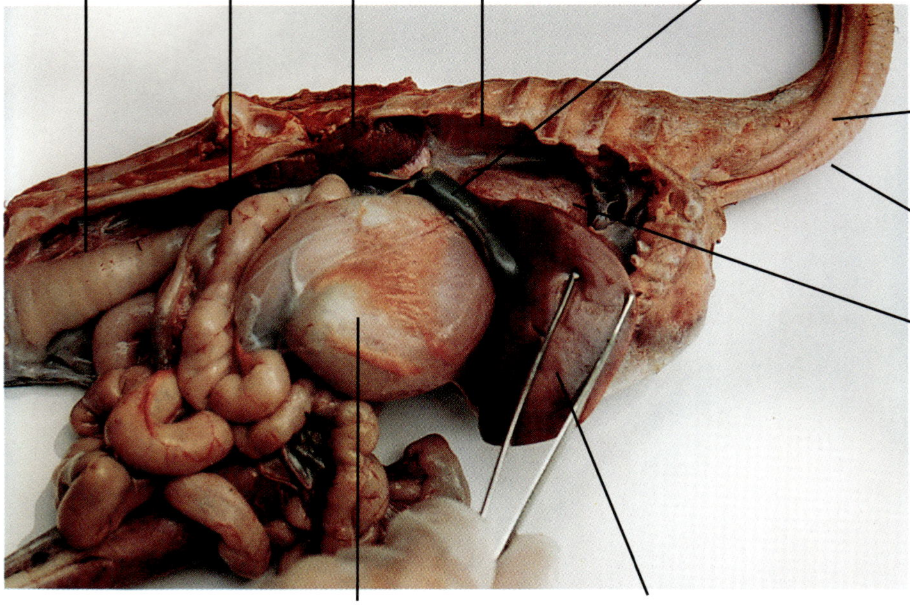

Plate 4.9 - Abdominal cavity of 2-month-old emu chick, side view. Note prominent gall bladder and large size of gizzard.

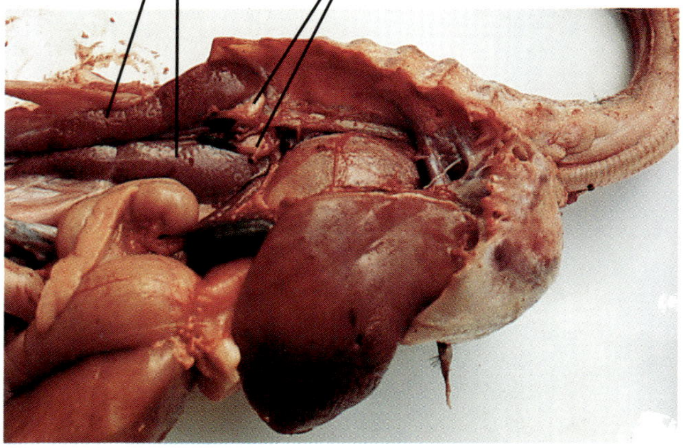

Plate 4.10 - View of kidneys with testes at top.

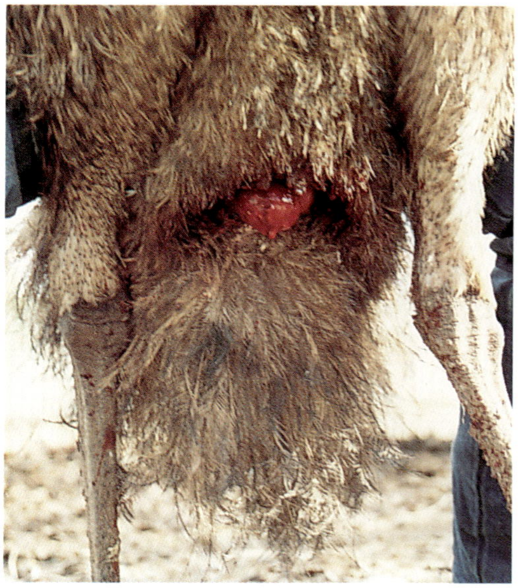

Plate 13.2 - Female emu with prolapsed oviduct.

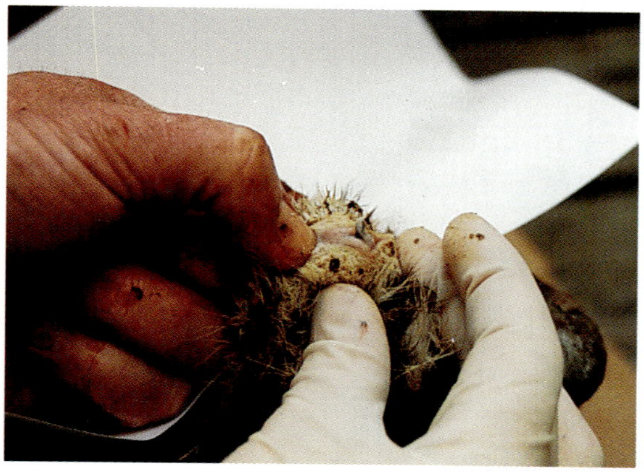

Plate 5.3 - Clearly visible sexual organ (phallus) of male emu chick.

Sexing emus at different ages

Plates 5.3 - 5.7

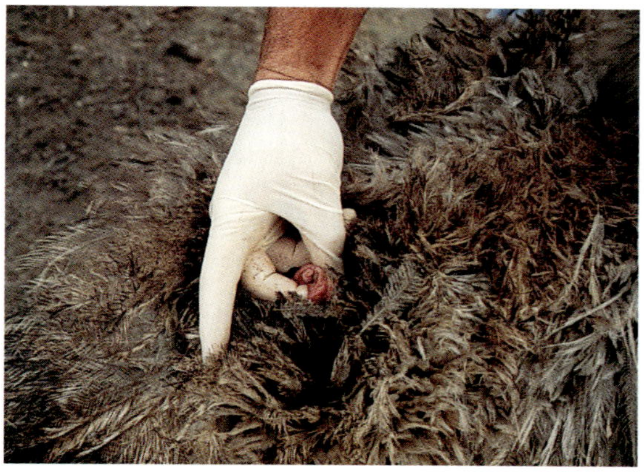

Plate 5.4 - Sexual organ of 8 month male, showing slight corkscrew twist.

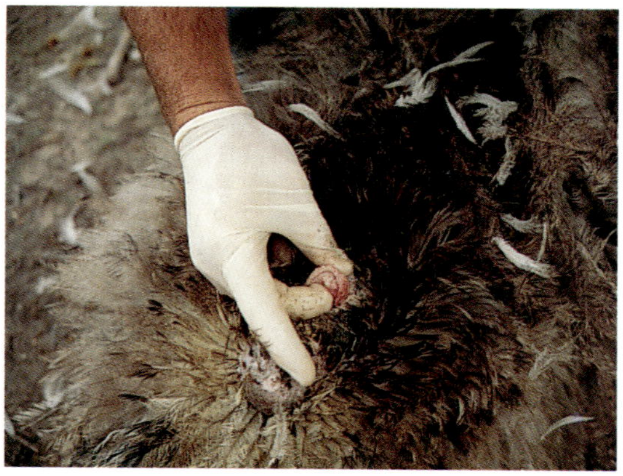

Plate 5.6 - Sex organ of yearling female - small protuberance.

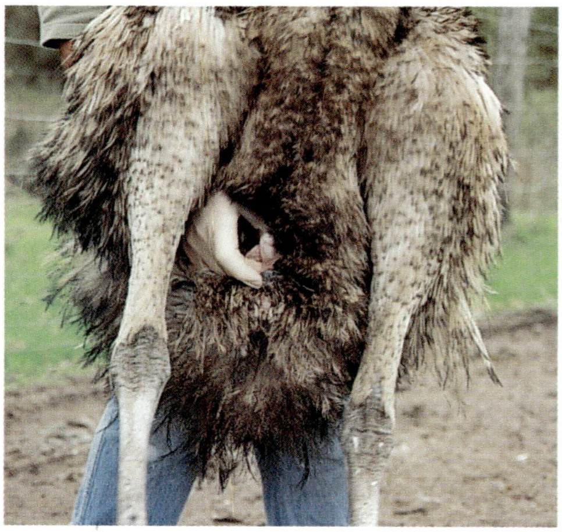

Plate 5.5 - Sexual organ (phallus) of fully grown male emu.

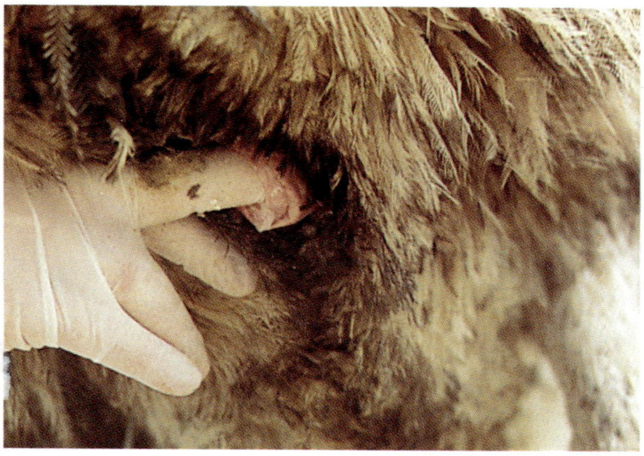

Plate 5.7 - Sex organ of adult female.

yellowish color, probably from the action of bile, and is very tough and elastic in order to withstand all the grinding which takes place in it. Note that both the entrance and exit of the gizzard are on its upper surface, making it a "cul-de-sac" of sorts - necessary to retain stones for grinding, but also making impactions possible. Fortunately, emus do not as a rule often suffer from impactions, as they are not such indiscriminate eaters as some of the other members of the ratite family. Also, an emu's gizzard is smaller and rounder than the elongated gizzard of the rhea.

4. **Duodenum** - This is the first part of the small intestine. It exits from the top part of the gizzard and forms a U-shaped loop which is held together by thin, translucent membranes. The **pancreas** (which secretes digestive enzymes) is held by membranes in this loop, and the membranes also contain a network of blood vessels. The pancreas is usually cream colored to pale yellow, and has "sharp" edges like the liver. (Looks like smooth fat).

5. **Jejunum** - Second part of small intestine, extending as far as the diverticulum.

6. **Diverticulum** - This small nodule is the remnant of the yolk sac, which shrinks rapidly as its nutrients are absorbed so that at the age of about 3 weeks, only this diverticulum remains. It is about the size of half a pea, and generally bright yellow in color in the young chick.

7. **Ileum** - The third and final part of the small intestine. It extends from the diverticulum to the juncture of the ceca. Not to be confused with the ILIUM, which is a part of the pelvic bone (see **Fig. 4.1** Emu Skeleton.)

8. **Juncture of small intestine with large intestine** - this is also the site of the juncture of the ceca.

9. **Paired ceca** - Birds differ from mammals in that instead of having one cecum, they have 2 ceca. The function is basically the same: bacterial digestion (fermentation) of fiber. The emu's ceca are not very long compared with those of the ostrich or rhea. Each cecum in the adult emu is about $2\frac{1}{4}$" (6cm) in length, compared with the rhea whose ceca are 32" and 38" respectively (80 cm and 95 cm.) In the emu as in the rhea, one cecum is sometimes a little shorter than the other, but this is not as noticeable

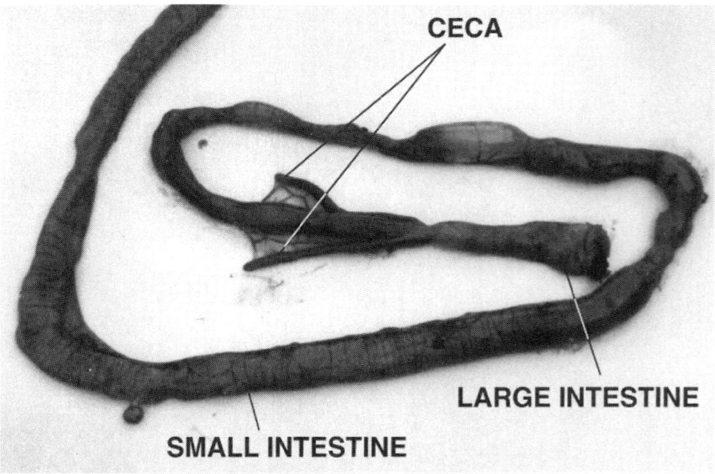

Plate 4.6 - Part of intestine of emu chick, showing position of small intestine, large intestine, and ceca.

since the ceca are short to begin with. Also, the emu's ceca are fairly narrow, resembling an earthworm, whereas the rhea has thick, bubbly ceca. An emu's ceca more closely resembles those of a chicken than those of an ostrich or rhea, showing that one should never assume that just because birds may look similar on the outside they have similar anatomical functions. There are always some species differences. Emu ceca are usually darker (green) at their tips.

10. **Colon** - The colon and ceca together make up the large intestine of birds. Absorption of water mainly takes place in the colon. The colon is fairly short and quite wide, usually occupies a position just under the kidneys in the bird, and opens into the cloaca.

11. **Cloaca** - This is the common chamber into which not only the digestive tract opens, but also the reproductive tracts (oviduct in females, sperm ducts in males) and ureters (from kidneys).

12. **Anus** - The "vent", or opening of the digestive tract to the outside for the elimination of waste products. Copulating and egg-laying takes place via the same hole. The anus is surrounded by a thick ring of contractile tissue which has many folds, allowing for plenty of expansion during defecation or egg-laying.

4.5 MAJOR ORGANS

It is important to know the relative positions and sizes of the major organs in the emu, so that if a bird becomes injured in different places one will have a good idea about which body structures are close to the site of the injury and might therefore also be affected. It is interesting to note, however, that all the organs are located in places where they are the most protected by the bird's strong skeletal structure - the kidneys under the fused pelvis/synsacrum, for instance, the lungs up under the thoracic part of the spinal column, and the heart nestling in the bowl-shaped sternum. The large liver is of course protected by the rib cage. Again, the structures shown are as viewed in a 3- to 4-month old emu, but the adult body is very much the same. The main difference in the adult bird would be the growth and development of the reproductive system, notably the oviduct in the female, as described in **Section 8.2** and **Fig. 8.1**.

As shown in **Fig 4.4**, the major organs are as follows:

1. **Brain**, encased in the skull which is quite thick.

2. Beginning of **spinal cord**, which runs from the brain all the way down the spinal column, encased in and protected by it. (The rest of the spinal cord is not shown.)

3. **Eyeball** - note large size, especially compared with size of brain, which shows how greatly the bird relies on its vision. (Two eyes together are larger than brain).

Chick hatching process

Plates 10.6 - 10.10

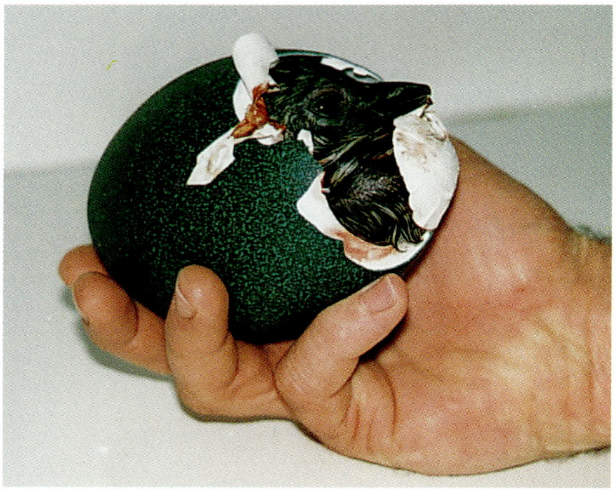

Plate 10.6 - Chick has opened shell.

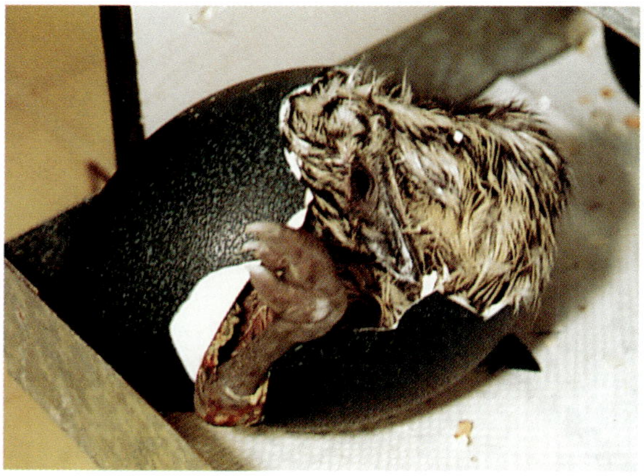

Plate 10.7 - Chick pushing hard against egg.

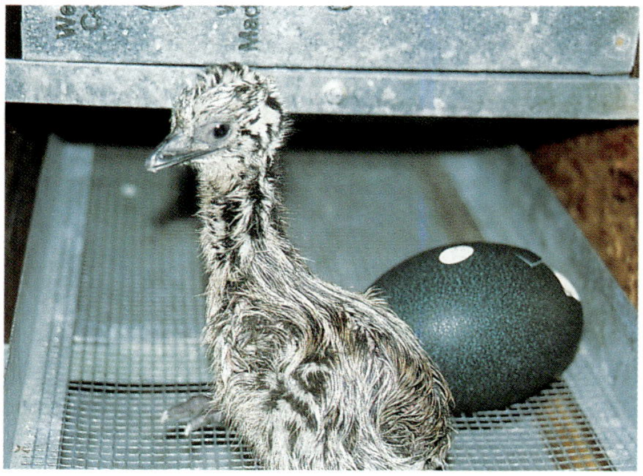

Plate 10.9 - Hatch complete; next egg just pipped.

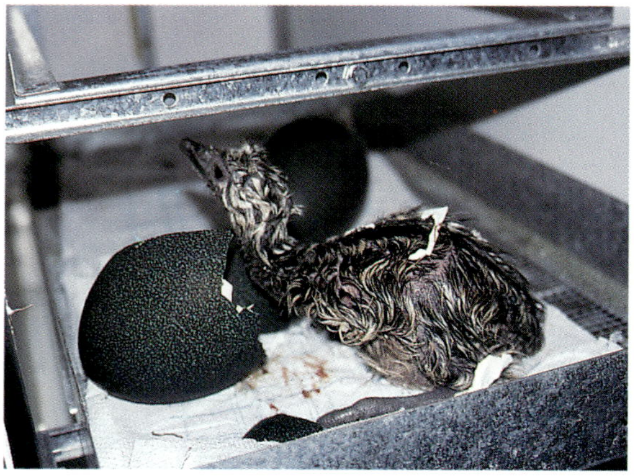

Plate 10.8 - Wet chick just crawled out of egg.

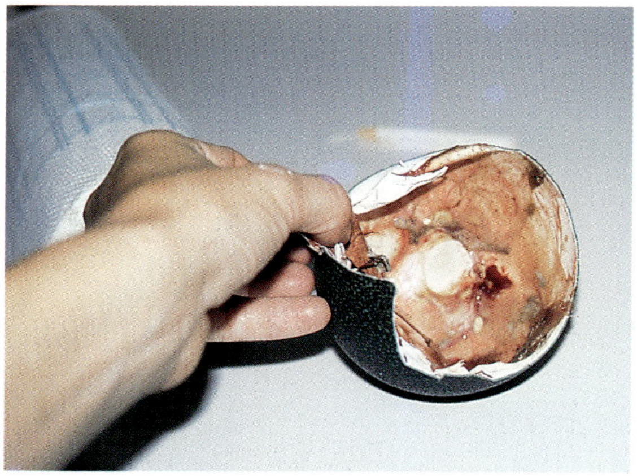

Plate 10.10 - Inner shell membrane and (vascular) chorio-allantois clearly visible in shell remnant from recently hatched chick.

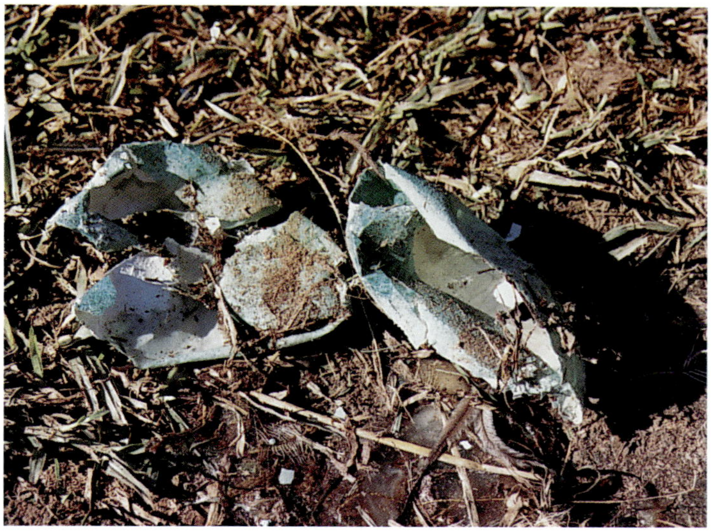

Plate 13.3
Soft-Shelled eggs.

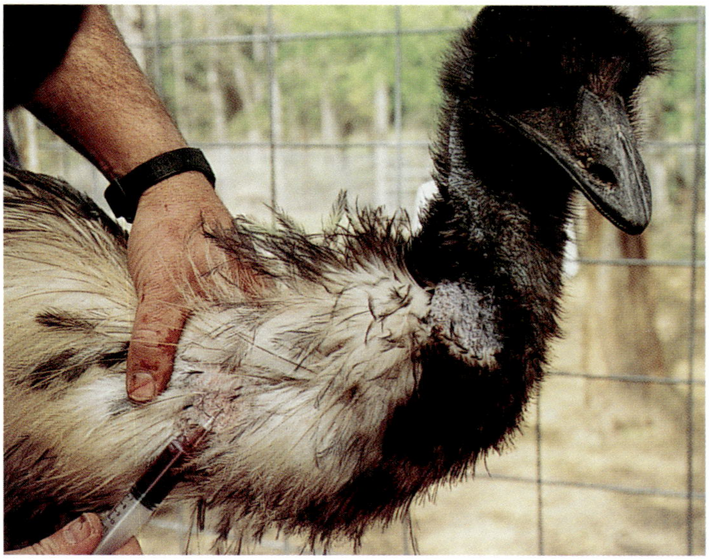

Plate 14.8
Drawing blood from jugular vein of emu.

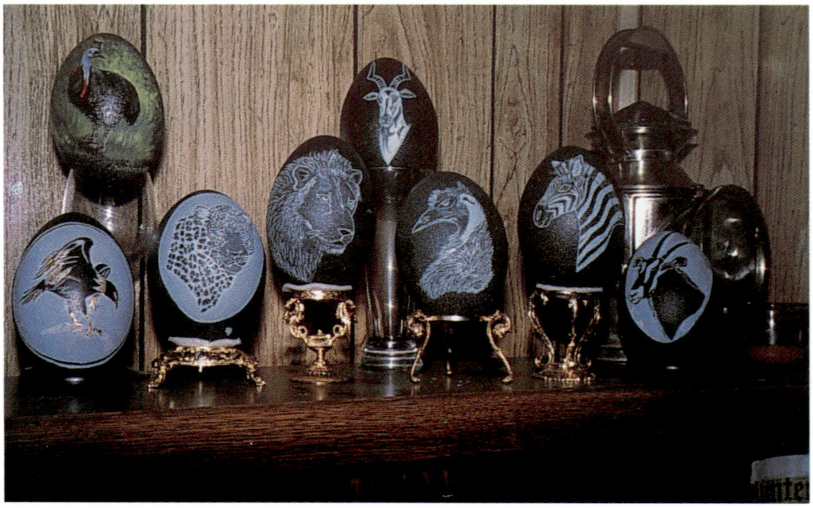

Plate 15.1
Decorated eggs.

4. **Nasal cavity**. Note the slanting tube that connects the nasal cavity to the roof of the mouth. The two nasal cavities are separated by a very thin septum (as are the two eyes), and each has a tube that culminates in the roof of the mouth, in the form of a small slit. These slits are useful for determining whether or not the nostrils are clogged up in upper respiratory infections, as described in **Section 14.6**.

5. **Opening of the trachea** (windpipe) in the bottom of the mouth. A sensitive reflex mechanism causes this opening to close completely at the slightest touch. This helps to ensure that food, water and foreign matter does not get into the trachea and contaminate the lungs. The small, triangular TONGUE is situated just in front of this opening.

6. **Trachea (windpipe.)** A fairly rigid white tube (in contrast to the esophagus which is completely soft, pliable and expandable) with rings of cartilage down its length for strength and support. This ensures that air can always pass freely through the trachea to and from the lungs. The esophagus lies dorsal to the trachea and slightly to the right of the trachea.

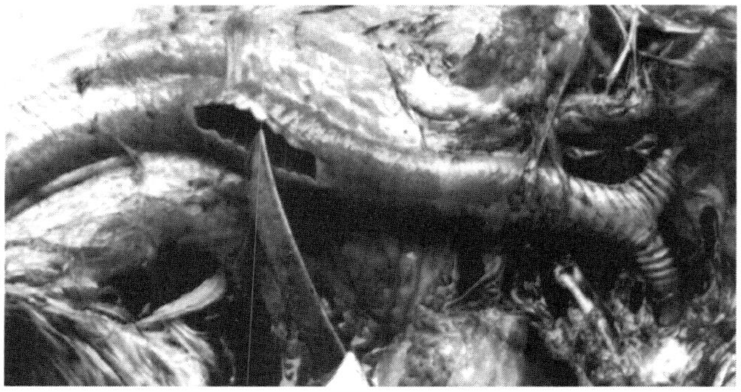

Plate 4.7 - Normal appearance of the opening in the trachea (adult emu).

7. **Smooth line down front of trachea**. In adult birds there is an opening here, presumably for making adult sounds (grunting in males, drumming in females) by forcing air through the hole in the trachea into an air sac. Possibly this hole starts to develop at about a year old, since this is when the chick's voice changes from whistling to the adult sounds. In the adult, the slit is about ½" wide and has somewhat jagged edges. (See **Plate 4.7**)

8. **Place where trachea divides into 2 bronchi**, which run on either side of the esophagus to the lungs.

9. **Lung**, which when healthy is a bright coral-pink color. Its texture is spongy. The two lungs lie next to each other, up against the thoracic vertebrae and at the very top of the rib cage.

10. **Heart**, part of which is covered by the liver.

11. **Liver** - has 2 main lobes, but the left lobe is somewhat smaller and subdivided. The gizzard lies between these two lobes and protrudes out

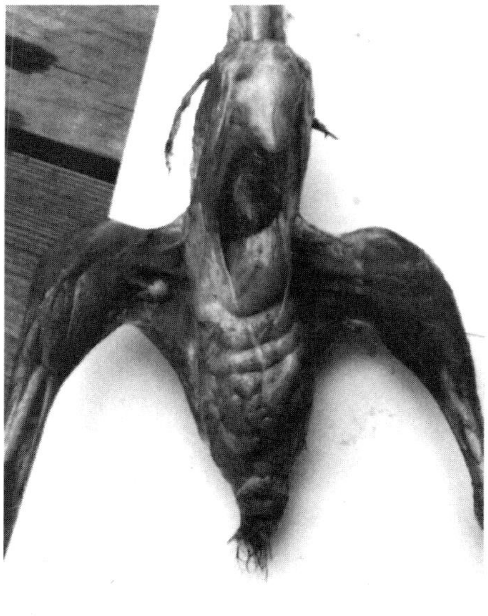

Plate 4.8 - Ventral view of emu showing consecutive positioning of sternum, liver, gizzard and intestine.

of them like a rosebud between two petals. A healthy liver is usually a reddish-brown color. When there is a lot of fat in the diet, the liver may have a more yellowish color. Its edge can be felt on a live bird by GENTLY palpating the belly beyond the edge of the sternum.

12. **Gall bladder** - attached to the inside of one of the lobes of the liver. Dark green in color, since it contains dark green bile, a fluid which is manufactured in the liver, stored in the gall bladder and used to help emulsify fats in the gut for digestion. Bile is secreted into the duodenum from both gall bladder and liver via short BILE DUCTS.

13. **Spleen** - also reddish-brown like the liver, but usually a darker color. A somewhat spongy sausage-like structure, lying along the top of the gizzard and proventriculus. Possibly used in lymphocyte production and the final destruction of blood cells.

14. One of the two **testes**, if the bird is a male. (The other testis is in the same position by the other kidney.) If the bird is a female, the ovary will be in approximately the same position, but on the left side only. A (white) sperm duct runs from each testis to the cloaca, along the same path as the ureters.

15. One of the two **kidneys**. The kidney has 3 lobes, and its color is usually a muddy chocolate-brown.

16. **Ureter** - a white tube that runs from kidney to cloaca and carries excretory products (uric acid) to the cloaca for elimination via the vent. There are two ureters (one running from each kidney) and they lie in between the two kidneys, just under the vertebral column.

17. **End part of ureter**, which empties into the cloaca.

Note: The transparent membranes that encase the gut and some of the organs are not usually fat-laden in the emu as they are in the chicken and many other bird species. Instead, they are thin and translucent. When a fat layer begins to develop in the full-grown bird, it is found just under the skin and is thickest over the area of the back. It is a very oily fat.

Some of the membranes found inserted between organs are no doubt AIR SACS, which are extensions of the bird's respiratory system. The emu, in common with other birds, has no DIAPHRAGM as such.

4.6 THE NEWLY HATCHED EMU CHICK

In order to detect problems or abnormalities in an animal, one must first know what is normal. The newly hatched emu chick is different in a few respects from an older bird, and a representation of its internal organs, their structure and position, is shown in **Fig. 4.5**. If it becomes necessary to autopsy a dead emu chick, the diagram will help in the identification of the structures seen. The diagram shows the chick in cross-section, lying on its left side with the right leg completely removed. For the sake of clarity, the only bones shown are the spine and the top part of the pelvis (22, the ilium). Also the gut has been shortened. The incision for dissection can be made at the lower end of the sternum (not shown, but it is the bowl-shaped bone in which the heart (14) lies). A blunt-nosed pair of scissors is adequate for dissection, since there is less chance of puncturing anything than with a scalpel or blade. The picture is much clearer if one can avoid spilling blood or gut or yolk contents into the stomach cavity. The incision is made ventrally towards the anus (12), and can then be widened by cutting across. The ribs, which encase the liver and other organs in the front half of the bird (thorax) are quite soft, being more cartilage than bone in the newly hatched chick, and they can be cut across with the scissors in order to get a better view inside and enlarge the opening.

In the newly hatched chick **(Fig. 4.5)**, the structures are as follows:

Breathing Apparatus

1. Opening of trachea in bottom of mouth - closes on reflex when touched.

2. Trachea (windpipe) - white tube with stiff cartilaginous rings around it.

3. Trachea splits on either side of esophagus to form 2 bronchi which go to the lungs.

4. One of the two lungs, situated up against spinal column. Healthy lungs are a bright coral-pink color and have a spongy texture.

Digestive System

5. Esophagus

6. Proventriculus (glandular stomach.)

7. Gizzard or ventriculus (muscular stomach)

8. Duodenum (first part of small intestine.)

9. YOLK SAC, covered with very vascular membrane. (Large at birth, shrunk to about 2½" x 2" in normal 4-day-old chick whose birth weight was 314g.)

10. Ceca. At their point of attachment, the small intestine ends and the large intestine begins.

11. Colon

12. Anus (vent)

13. Navel, through which the yolk sac was pulled into body cavity prior to hatch. By hatching, navel should be closed.

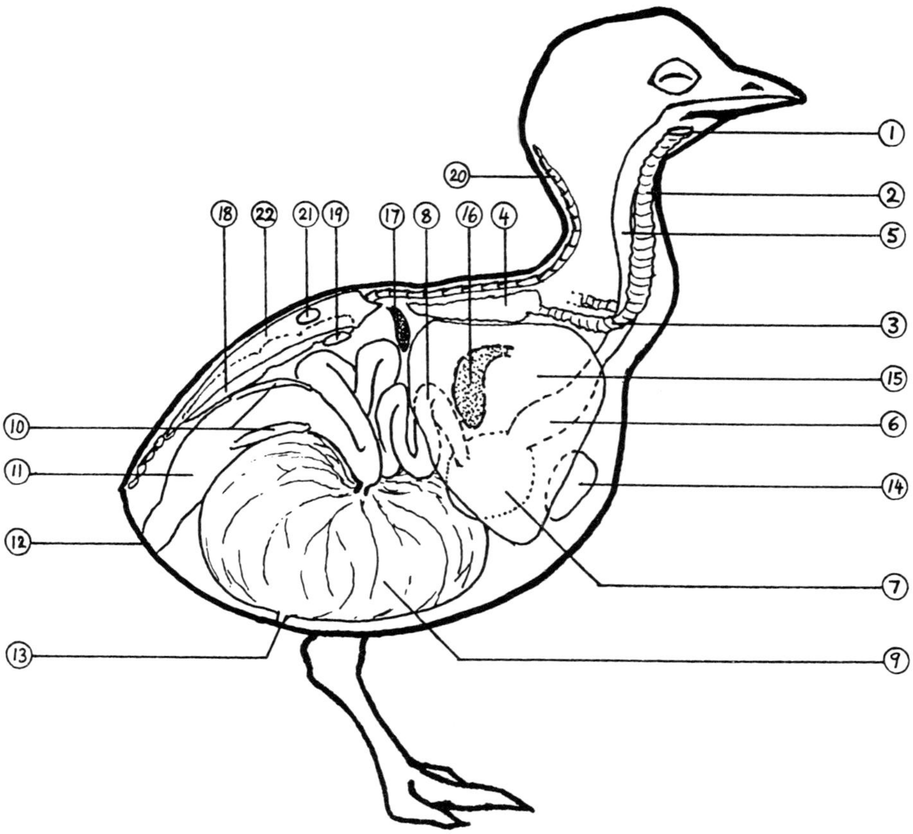

Fig. 4.5 -Representation of gut and major organs in newly hatched emu chick.

Other Major Organs

14. Heart

15. Liver

16. Gall bladder - a dark green elongated sac, attached to one of the inside lobes of the liver. It contains dark green bile, which may also have stained the areas around it (liver and nearest parts of gut). The staining is normal. Length in 4-day-old chick: 2cm. ($^3\!/_4$").

17. Spleen - a dark brownish-red sac-like structure, somewhat spongy in section.

18. One of the two kidneys, which lie next to each other up against the synsacrum (fused inside part of pelvic bone). Each is quite long, sausage-shaped and divided into 3 lobes. The two ureters (not shown) are white tubes lying between the kidneys which run downwards from the kidneys toward the anus and empty into the cloaca (final chamber of gut), where the waste products are excreted as semi-solid white uric acid.

19. One of the two testes, if the bird is a male, each lying at top of a kidney. A female will have the beginnings of an ovary, on the left side only but in approximately the same position. Confirm findings by vent-sexing (**Section 5.2**).

Bones

20. Spinal column

21. Hip joint, where head of femur joins pelvic girdle

22. Ilium (top part of pelvic bone. Other parts of pelvic bone not shown.)

Differences between new hatchling and older chick

The main difference between a chick that has just hatched and an older chick is of course the presence of the yolk sac (9), which makes the chick's belly appear quite round and fat. Since the yolk sac contains all of the chick's food and it has not eaten yet, the gizzard (7) is relatively small. By contrast, the area around the point of attachment of the yolk sac to the gut is usually filled with yolk material which may vary in color from dirty yellow to dirty green. The green color is no doubt due to the secretion of BILE into the gut from the gall bladder (16), which stores bile after it has been manufactured in the liver (15).

Since the newly hatched chick still has a large amount of yolk to use up, and since yolk contains a lot of fat, it is not surprising that in the new hatchling the gall bladder is rather large and prominent. Bile (from the gall bladder) is a dark green liquid which aids in the digestion of fat, by acting as an emulsifying agent. The liver itself is a lot more yellow in color in the newly-hatched chick (compared with older birds) due to the large amount of fat metabolized.

As the chick grows, both the gizzard (7) and the proventriculus (6) will also grow, and the yolk sac will shrink as its contents get used up. By the time the chick is 3 weeks old, the yolk sac will have shrunk to a small nodule about the size of half a pea, attached to the small intestine. It is no longer attached at the navel (13). The nodule is usually quite a bright yellow color. During the first 3 weeks, the gizzard will gradually have grown to replace the position in the chick's abdomen formerly occupied by the yolk sac. Thus, in a month-old or older chick, the "hard" belly which can be felt when picking up the chick after it has just eaten is not yolk sac, but gizzard. It will feel much softer a few hours after the meal, as the food is digested.

CHAPTER 5

Sexing the Emu

The sexing of different species of birds is commonly done by one of these methods:

• Vent-sexing, by feel and/or examination of sex organs just inside the vent.

• Observation of secondary sex characteristics (usually only possible in sexually mature birds) e.g. different coloring in ostriches, different sounds in emus, different combs and plumage in chickens

• Endoscopy, or surgical sexing - an endoscope is inserted into the bird under mild anesthesia in order to view the testes or ovary.

• Study of differences in male/female chromosomes in tissue or blood samples. (This would be a good area for research in emus, as it is non-invasive and does not depend on age.)

Emus, unlike many other bird species, do not display much visible difference between males and females. For this reason it is important to become skilled at "sexing" them, so that mistakes can be avoided when buying or selling birds. This is a relatively easy task on tame adult birds, but may be more difficult on younger birds not only because the sexual organs are still immature but also because young birds tend to offer a lot more resistance to handling. The only effective way to learn is by a lot of practice, on many birds of different ages and with an experienced person to help clarify the results if possible. The photographs (see color section) will help show visible differences, but sexing by "feel" will come with experience.

5.1 SEXING THE ADULT BIRD

The adult bird can be held in the normal way with one hand around the chest while standing behind it, leaving the other hand free to manually sex the bird. The finger is inserted into the cloaca and the organ is everted by rolling it out with the thumb against the forefinger. Using a (non-sterile) latex glove ensures comfort for the emu and protection for your skin from the strong, permeating odor of the emu's cloaca. Be prepared for a little resistance from the bird, and resume sexing only when he is standing quietly again, to avoid injury. An assistant to help hold the bird can be useful. The photos of the adult birds (**Plates 5.5 & 5.7** of color section) show typically the size and shape of the organs. Obviously some variations will occur.

In the adult male emu the sex organ (phallus) is hard all the time as it is supported by "cartilage". The organ is generally around $2\frac{1}{2}$" long and about 2" at the base, tapering to about $\frac{1}{2}$" at the tip.

The adult female has a small clitoris which feels soft, compared with the male's organ. It is in exactly the same position where the phallus can be found in the male. The clitoris will vary in size from about $\frac{3}{4}$" long to virtually nothing, and is rarely thicker than $\frac{1}{2}$".

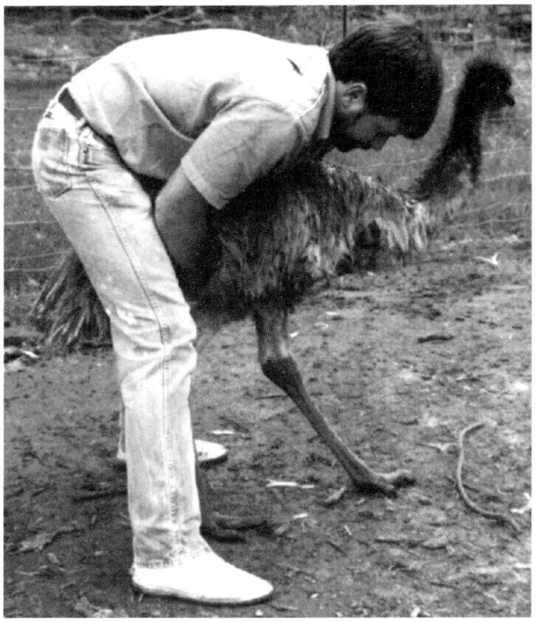

Plate 5.1 - Sexing the bird in a standing position.

5.2 SEXING THE CHICK

To sex an emu chick, first grasp the two legs and, holding them firmly together, lay the bird gently on its back. Then place thumb and forefinger on either side of the bird's vent and with a gentle kneading motion, evert the cloaca until the organ can be clearly seen. Birds from a few days to several months old can be sexed in this way. The only difference is in the amount of assistance needed to hold an older, stronger bird; while it is possible for one person to sex a ten- or eleven-month old bird in this way (as shown in **Plate 5.2**) it is definitely easier with at least one assistant. By everting the cloaca rather than inserting a finger into the bird, there is less danger of harm to the bird, especially in very young chicks.

Emu chicks can be sexed successfully from one or two days old. However, occasionally chicks are encountered whose organ has a very confusing shape. These are best left for a few months to develop further, and can then be re-sexed. There really is no noticeable "cartilage" or harder tissue in young chicks so it is more difficult to differentiate between the sexes. The male generally has a larger organ, lighter in color (can appear almost white) and with a corkscrew twist to one side. The top of the organ has a noticeable fold or opening. The female organ is generally smaller with a "rosier" color and has a smaller tip to it. Some females will have virtually no clitoris, or only a small protrusion as big as a pen tip. The female sex organ, unlike that of the male, does not grow or change much from birth to maturity.

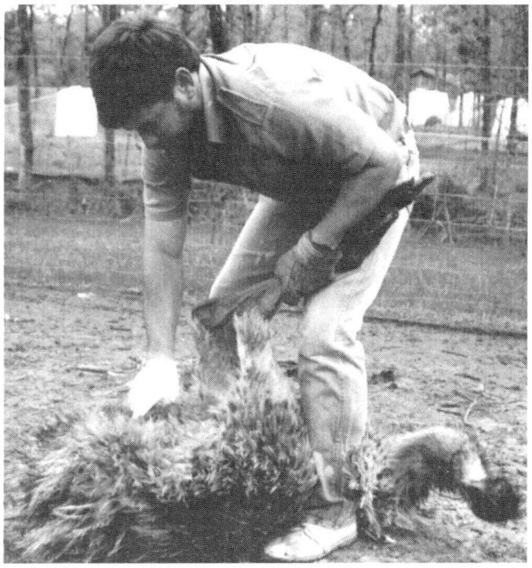

Plate 5.2 - Laying bird down to sex it.

Caution must be exercised when sexing very young chicks. Unless the birds are going to be sold and it is necessary to sex them, it is better to wait until they are older. Inexperienced or rough sexing of a bird can hurt it.

5.3 SEXUAL DEVELOPMENT AND CHARACTERISTICS

The birds develop very little sexually in their first year. Although they grow almost to their full height in this time, not much development will usually have taken place in their sex organs. The greatest change seems to occur from about 12 to 20 months in most birds, with males obviously showing the greatest physical change as the phallus grows to full size in a few months.

At about 10 to 14 months old, most birds also stop chirping/whistling and start to make adult sounds instead. Grunting will be heard instead of cheeping and soon after, the female's transitory grunting changes to a deeper drumming sound. The female's throat sac is still developing at this time, and therefore it is not uncommon to hear sounds somewhere in between grunting and drumming. By the time she is around two years old, the sound should have changed to a more guttural drumming, easily distinguished from the grunting of the males. Of course, all these time factors are averages and obviously there will be exceptions where birds develop at a faster or slower rate. This is not abnormal, as all animals (and humans) will vary somewhat in how soon they become sexually mature.

Many mature female emus make their deep, rhythmical drumming sound all through the year; others only during breeding season. There is often more drumming heard in the evening and night, as well as early morning, than at other times of day during breeding season. For some reason the approach of colder weather or thunderstorms also often causes an increase in drumming. The female can usually drum in two pitches: a higher and faster stuttering sound often heard when the female is caught and handled, and the much deeper, more resonant booming that sounds like tribal drums in the wilderness.

A strutting female with a large, pendulous throat sac is most often a younger bird (2-to 3-year-old). As females get older these sacs appear to get drawn up, and it becomes more rare to see the sac drop down. When it is let down, it is usually only for short periods, when the female is strutting.

While there are many variations of shades of blue on the neck, amount of "hair" on the head and other such distinguishing characteristics among different emus, these differences have not been found to be sex-related. There is no known way of visibly telling males from females, other than by observation of the movement of the throat sac in mature breeders when sounds are made. (If several emus are together in one pen and one of them drums, it can be difficult to tell which one made the sound unless the bird's throat sac is seen vibrating.) An experienced person may be able to make an educated guess as to sexes in a pen of mature breeders which are not making any sounds, based on the fact that the female's throat sac often hangs like a dewlap on her chest before and during breeding season, as well as the friendly behavior of many of the males. However, since the male and female both fluff out their neck feathers and strut around during breeding season, an older female with a smaller "dewlap" may be mistaken for a male, and a male with longer chest feathers may look like a female. If no sounds are being made, the only way to know sexes with certainty is by manual sexing.

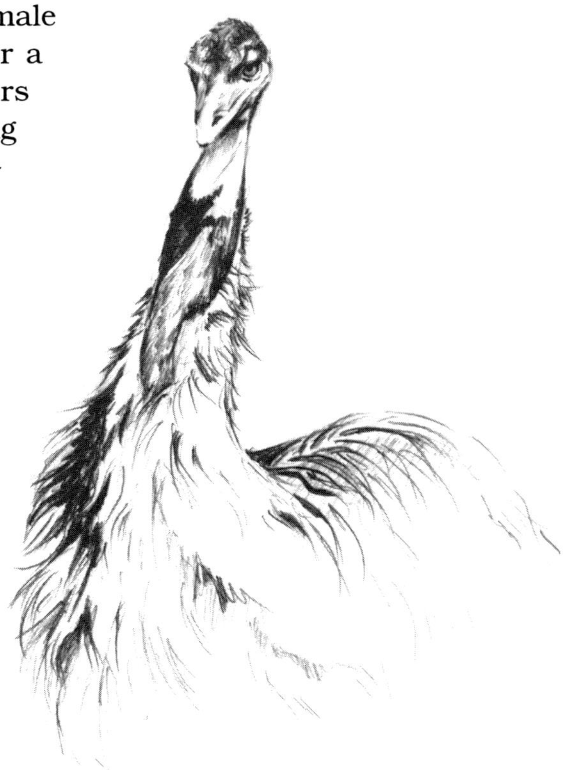

CHAPTER 6

Nutrition

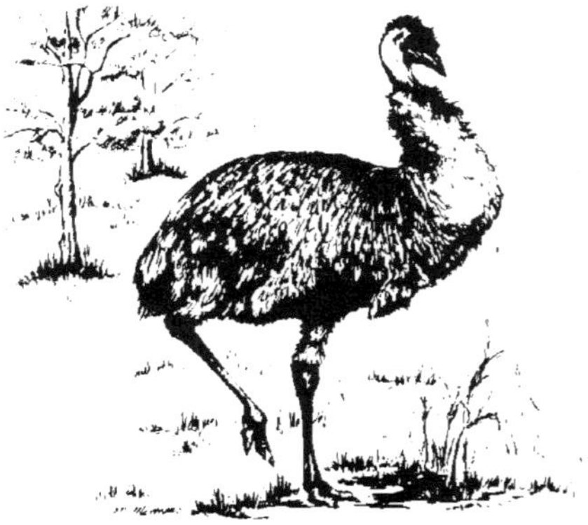

6.1 INTRODUCTION

Every farmer has to learn as much as he possibly can about the specific dietary needs of the animals he is farming. This is because he is the one providing their food, as well as restricting their movement in search of food by means of fences and pens. If his animals do not grow, thrive and reproduce as they should, the farmer's livelihood suffers too.

Good nutrition is a vital part of good management technique, not only to keep animals growing and reproducing but also to maintain good health and resistance to disease.

While a lot of research has been done on the more common domesticated farm animals such as cattle, pigs, poultry etc., as well as pet animals such as cats, dogs and caged birds, this is not the case with the emu as it has not been farmed for very long. In the quest for the optimum emu diet, one can get a good starting insight by finding the answers to the following questions:

1. What does the gut of the emu look like, and how might this relate to what its diet should be?

2. What does the emu eat in the wild?

3. Based on similarities in feeding habits, structure of gut and signs of nutritional deficiencies, what bird/animal for which a commercially prepared feed is already available, does the emu most resemble? What are significant differences between the species?

4. What types of feed have already been used for emus with LONG-TERM good results? What diets have not worked well?

In the sections that follow, these questions will be dealt with as fully as our present knowledge allows, remembering that there may be points that have been overlooked due to lack of information. However, one has to start somewhere.

6.2 RELATIONSHIP OF DIET TO DIGESTIVE SYSTEM

"Dietary needs" and "nutritional needs" of an animal are not the same thing. Although most animals have the same basic nutritional needs, in terms of proteins, fats, carbohydrates, vitamins and minerals, the food sources that they can use to meet those needs can be extremely different. This is because every single species of animal or bird has a digestive system adapted specifically to its kind of diet. Therefore, something that one animal can utilize as food, another cannot.

For instance, cattle do not need a source of B-vitamins in their diet. This is not because their bodies do not need B-vitamins (they do), but because the beneficial bacteria in the rumen (compartmented stomach) synthesize enough B-vitamins to meet all body needs. It is the presence of these "good bacteria" that ensure that cattle can thrive on a diet that is chiefly grass or hay - undigestible fiber to many other species.

By looking at the gut system of an animal, it is possible to place the animal into one of three broad categories:

1. **Herbivores** - utilize mainly grass and other less easily digested plant material for food. In order to break the fiber (cellulose) down, beneficial bacteria are needed in the gut. Because it takes time for the fermenting action of bacteria to do their work, a very LONG gut is needed, along with extra compartments where micro-organisms can thrive without being moved down through the gut by its peristaltic movements. In ruminants such as cattle and sheep, a compartmented stomach provides this "fermentation vat". In other herbivores such as horses and rabbits, the **cecum** is large and well developed, and provides such a place for fiber fermentation since it is a "cul-de-sac" of sorts. Birds, unlike mammals, have **two ceca**, and the function appears to be the same: digestion of fiber. Some seed-eating birds have very rudimentary ceca, as fiber does not form a significant part of their diet. Others, like the rhea and ostrich, have rather long, large and bubbly-looking ceca which is in keeping with their utilization of grass as part of their diet.

2. **Omnivores** - utilize food both of plant and animal origin, and total length of gut compared with body length is less than in herbivores since the animal relies less on bacterial digestion. Higher quality plant material than grass/hay is normally utilized. Length of ceca in omnivorous birds is variable, but generally the ceca are shorter and smaller than in more herbivorous birds. Chickens, turkeys and emus fit into this category.

3. **Carnivores** - utilize chiefly meat as the food source, and therefore generally have a yet shorter gut in comparison to body length and rudimentary cecum or ceca. Time of food passage is generally shortest in carnivores since animal proteins take a lot less time to digest than fibrous plant matter.

Note that this is a very general way of looking at dietary needs for different animals - there are many animals that fit between two of these categories, as shown in **Fig. 6.1** . However, going from the general to the specific helps in establishing the "big picture". Specifics can be narrowed down later.

The digestive tract of the emu (refer to **Fig. 4.3** in Anatomy chapter) indicates that it is basically an omnivore, for two reasons:

1. Although ceca are present (showing some fiber digestion probably takes

place) they are not very long or thick, compared with the ceca of more herbivorous ratites such as the rhea or ostrich.

2. The total length of gut compared with body length is much shorter than that of more herbivorous birds. In keeping with this, food also passes through the emu's gut rather quickly.

The time of food passage in an animal is related to the nature of its diet. For

HERBIVORES	**OMNIVORES**	**CARNIVORES**
feeding on plant material	feeding on plant and animal material	feeding on animal material
long digestive tract relative to body length	shorter digestive tract relative to body length	v. short digestive tract relative to body length

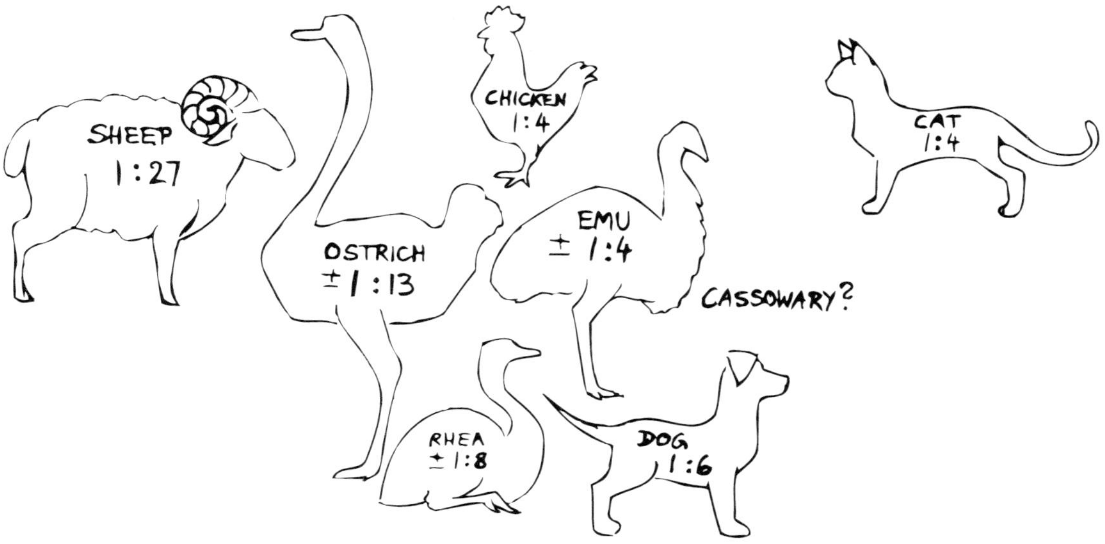

plenty of bacterial digestion (fermentation), allowing a lot of fiber to be used as a food source	some bacterial digestion but fiber not so well utilized as food source	little or no bacterial digestion

Fig. 6.1 - Diagram showing general relationship of gut length to body length, and how this relates to diet.

instance, in ruminants it takes 40 to 80 hours for food to pass through; horses, around 30 hours; ostrich, about 48 hours. All these animals are basically herbivorous. In the emu, by contrast, food takes 6-8 hours to pass through, indicating its more omnivorous diet. It also makes sense that the shorter the gut, the shorter the time of food passage - and the more efficient the gut has to be. For these reasons, the emu will make better use of good quality food whose nutrients are highly available, than food which contains large quantities of crude fiber and/or is less digestible.

6.3 DIET OF EMU IN THE WILD

Most texts agree that the emu is able to survive well in the wild on small quantities of a high-quality diet, including fruit, seeds, broad-leaved plants, shoots, flowers and the occasional insect or grub when available. Sources differ as to the bird's ability to digest fiber, but it is likely that some (bacterial) digestion of fiber takes place in the ceca, ileum and colon.

In seasons of plenty, the adult emu lays down a food reserve in the form of a thick layer of sub-cutaneous fat which is especially thick along the back. Emus may eat some grass, but it never forms the main part of their diet.

6.4 SIMILARITIES AND DIFFERENCES BETWEEN POULTRY AND EMUS

(a) Anatomy

Strange though it may seem, the gut of an emu more closely resembles that of a chicken than that of an ostrich or rhea, even though the latter two species are more closely related to it. However, when one considers the diet of a chicken - also an omnivore which like the emu feeds on seeds/grubs/greenery/insects - the similarity is perhaps not so remarkable after all.

The main differences between poultry and emus are the much larger SIZE of the emu, and the much longer GROWTH PERIOD. The emu reaches maturity after more than a year; the chicken, after a number of weeks. The emu also has much longer legs relative to body size; in this, the bird resembles the turkey more (or at least its wild counterpart). With this in mind, it would seem that a good chicken or turkey diet would be a good place to start from in the feeding of emus. To promote optimum skeletal growth during the long growth period, however, there could well be a need for higher levels of some vitamins, in particular those which promote growth - the B-vitamins. Mineral balances would need to be proportionately correct during the whole growth process to prevent any abnormalities, and protein levels probably should not be too high or this could promote too rapid a growth of body protein (muscle and organs) before the skeleton, slower-growing, was equipped to handle the heavier body weight. (This problem can also lead to deformities.)

Some turkey and poultry **starter** diets are designed to put as much weight on a bird in as little time as possible. This is obviously not desirable in the emu, and these high-protein starter diets should probably be avoided altogether unless "diluted" with greens or other low-protein feed.

(b) Deficiences

Deficiency symptoms in the emu chick compared with chickens/turkeys are remarkably similar. In all these species, deficiencies in one or more of the B- vitamins are the most common. **The B-vitamins** are:

Thiamine (B1)

Riboflavin (B2)

Niacin (nicotinic acid)

Pyridoxine (B6)

Pantothenic acid

Biotin

Choline

Folacin (folic acid)

Cyanocobalamin (B12)

Any deficiency symptoms seen in the first week after hatching are likely to be caused by a deficiency in the **breeder diet**, or some other stress at the time the hen laid that particular egg. Deficiencies seen after 2-3 weeks are probably caused by a poorly balanced **chick diet**, since by this time the chick has almost finished absorbing his yolk sac internally and is relying on the diet for his total nutritional needs.

Deficiencies noted are as follows:

1. **Head retraction/head weaving** - In pigeons, chickens and turkeys this condition is known as "polyneuritis" and is caused by a deficiency of THIAMINE (a B-vitamin). A similar condition occurs in emu chicks (**Plate 6.1**). Within the first day of hatching, the chick begins to "star-gaze" and may also chirp loudly and insistently, as well as experience frequent head tremors. After a while the head retracts backwards and weaves back and forth across the back. The chick may even sleep with its beak pointing upwards in this way. Sometimes the head retracts so far backwards that the chick topples over. In some (but not all) cases,the condition occurred in chicks from eggs that had had very high weight loss (close to 20%), suggesting that dehydration may have played a part, e.g. in failure to utilize properly the contents of the yolk sac, at least to begin with. **Treatment**: In all cases the symptoms seemed to lessen when the chick was placed outside for sunshine and exercise, and encouraged to drink.

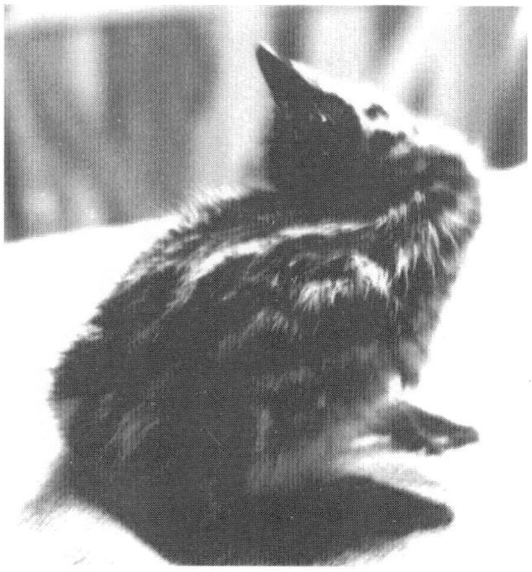

Plate 6.1 - Head retraction in day-old emu chick believed to be caused by thiamine deficiency.

Some cases were rehydrated by injecting several cc's of Lactated Ringer's Solution under the skin. (Tube-feeding liquids was found **not** to be a good idea as the head retraction can cause the small chick to get fluid down the trachea.) Most were injected with

Vitamin B Complex, some also with Vitamin E and Selenium. In all cases recovery was complete within 2 - 3 days.

It is also possible recovery would have been spontaneous if nothing had been done, but treatment with Vit.B Complex is recommended, since at the very least it will do no harm.

This condition has also been seen in an older chick with an acute infection. Tube-feeding with glucose, water and yeast reversed the problem very quickly, and the bird was also given a course of antibiotics (Amoxicillin). In poultry, thiamine deficiency symptoms in conjunction with certain infections is ascribed to the thiamine-destroying activity of some of these bacteria.

2. **Bent (bowed) legbones** - In ducks and turkeys, a deficiency in NIACIN (a B-vitamin) has been reported to cause bent legbones, differing from "rickets" (a calcium/phosphorus/Vitamin D3 imbalance) in that the bones are strong and hard, not soft and brittle. Emu chicks have been seen with this problem (**Plate 6.2**).

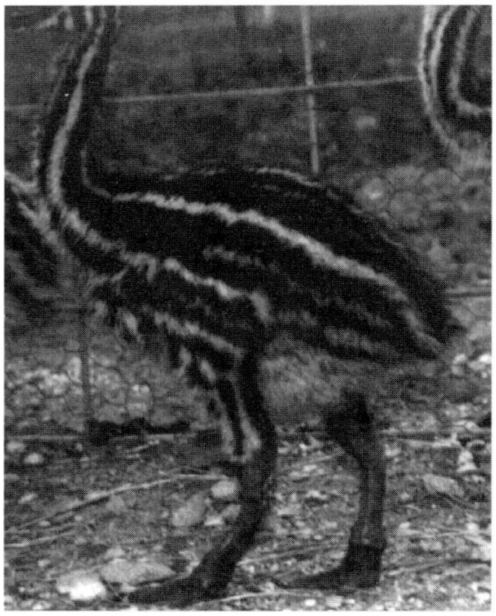

Plate 6.2 - Bent legbones in emu chick about 1 month old.

Although in some of the diets, the calcium/phosphorus ratio was not ideal, (in excess of 2:1), the fact that the bones seemed hard (no fractures were ever seen) and that the problem appeared worse in the bigger and faster-growing chicks (whose needs for B-vitamins would have been greater) seems to suggest that niacin deficiency was at least part of the problem. Perhaps it was aggravated by the less-than-perfect calcium/phosphorus ratio or insufficient Vit. D3. Enlarged hocks usually accompanies the bent legbones, and the most apparent bending is seen in the tarsometatarsus. Both tarsometatarsus and tibiotarsus may be shorter than normal, and mild "splaying" (see below) sometimes accompanies the condition, showing that in many cases, a deficiency in more than just one vitamin may be involved. Alternately, some birds begin to walk with toes pointed inwards like a bulldog. The thighs then become very rounded and heavily muscled. **Treatment**: If caught early enough, a change to a better diet with more B-vitamins may be beneficial, but unfortunately in many problems that involve the skeleton, at least some of the deformity remains, even if the bird is able to grow to adulthood. Prevention (through good nutrition) is the best "cure".

3. **"Splayed" leg** - In this condition, usually only one leg is affected and it may be either the right or the left leg. The affected leg faces outward at an angle rather

than pointing forward in the normal way, and as the bird grows, the condition worsens. Eventually, the bird is no longer able to get around and has to be killed. In one rare case, an emu compensated for his deformity by learning to center all

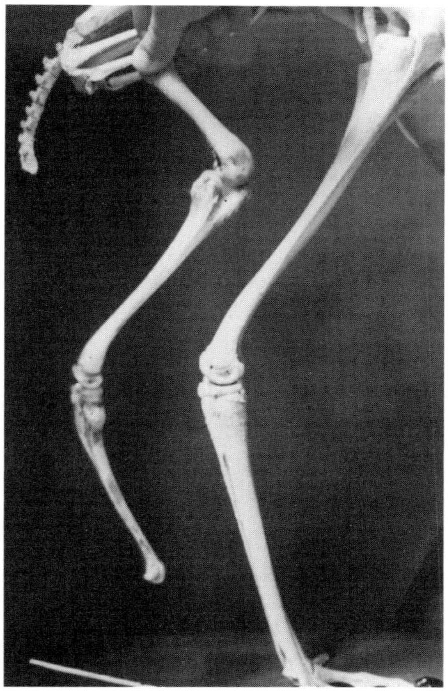

Plate 6.3 (a) - Abnormal leg bone (L), Normal leg bone (R), side view. Note bending and shortening of abnormal tarsometatarsus.

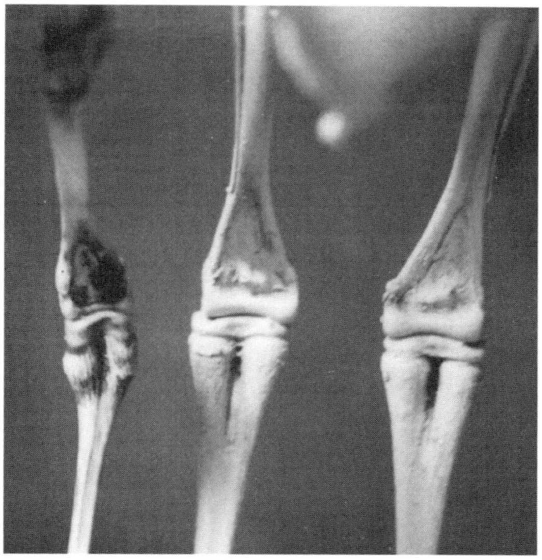

Plate 6.3 (b) - Abnormal legbone (L) compared with normal leg bones (R). View from front. Note abnormal top of tarsometatarsus. (birds were different ages).

his weight on one leg and hop on it, while the other, severely rotated, hung useless. Although the "healthy" leg grew very thick, it was abnormally short and the bird was stunted.

In chickens and turkeys, a "splayed-leg" condition (sometimes known as "perosis") can be due to a deficiency in one or more of the following: BIOTIN, CHOLINE, NIACIN and possibly FOLACIN (all B-vitamins) and the trace element MANGANESE. A deficiency of ZINC may also be a contributing factor.

Very often the problem appears to originate in the hip joint, in the emu cases seen. There seems to be more free movement in the joint than there should be, suggesting weak or overstretched tendons/ligaments, or possibly some kind of malformation in the joint itself such as too shallow a hip socket for the ball of the femur to fit into. (The latter occurs in dogs with hip dysplasia, and is an inherited tendency.) The hock joint also becomes enlarged and deformed. There may be some "corkscrew" type rotation in the tibiotarsus, as well as overall stunting in growth of the bird even though its appetite is good . The abnormal growth of the bones, in particular at the joints, means the tendons will also be in abnormal positions and, by exerting stresses and strains in the wrong places and at the wrong angles, the problem builds upon itself. **Treatment**: None found to date, except if the problem is caught very early, before too much damage has been done, and the diet is changed for the better. Unfortunately by the time the problem is noticed, some damage has already been done. In addition, the effects of a change of diet on the body are slow and may take several weeks, during which time irreparable damage may be done. Some surgical intervention has also been done on emu chicks (see **Section 14.4**) with limited success, but it is not usually economically feasible.

Having established that similar deficiency situations exist in emus as in turkeys or chickens, this shows that many of the dietary requirements for emus in terms of vitamins and minerals are going to be similar to those of poultry. All that remains is to find the correct balance of these nutrients for emus, both for growth, maintenance, "fattening" for slaughter, and reproduction. This is a fertile area for research, and many feed companies are now attempting to meet this challenge.

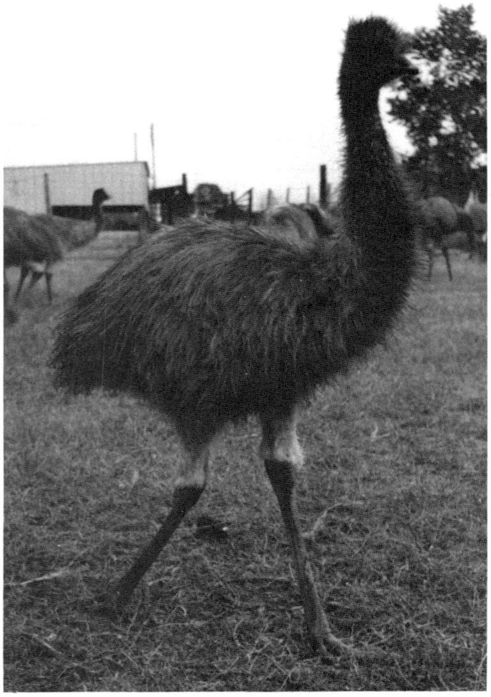

Plate 6.4 - Emu chick with "splayed" leg.

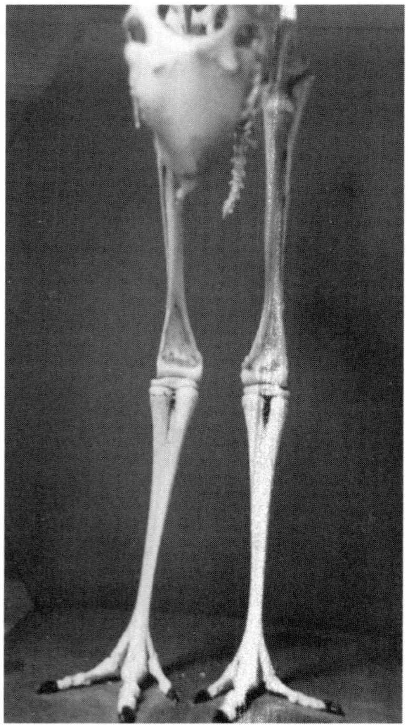

Plate 6.5 - Leg bones of normal 3-month old emu, front view.

6.5 THE "BALANCED" DIET.

It is important to remember that there is no single magic ingredient that an emu farmer can pour down the throat of his birds which will make them bigger, better and more productive. Good nutrition, as illustrated in **Fig. 6.2**, is a question of balance. How well the birds do will depend entirely on how closely one is able to approach the nutritional IDEAL for the emu, in terms of the relationships of all the nutrients required to each other.

Very broadly speaking, the largest portion of any animal's diet consists of CARBOHYDRATES, PROTEINS and FATS. These can all be used to provide ENERGY for various body functions. Proteins also have an important function in building up body tissue, in particular during growth and reproduction.

Just as important, but needed in smaller quantities are the VITAMINS. These are a group of organic substances which can vary greatly in chemical structure but which are needed in various enzyme systems for different body processes.

Finally, the body needs certain MINERALS, in particular for building up the skeleton. Some of these minerals are needed only in extremely small quantities, and these are known as TRACE ELEMENTS.

Some roles of different nutrients.

CARBOHYDRATES

Mainly used to provide energy. Complex carbohydrates such as **cellulose** (main constituent of "crude fiber") cannot be broken down by enzymes directly, but are broken down by the action of bacteria in the gut. **Starches** are more easily digested, especially by animals whose gut system is not well equipped for digestion by bacterial fermentation. During digestion, carbohydrates are broken down into "simple sugars" such as GLUCOSE, which can be readily assimilated by the body. (For this reason, animals which are in shock or otherwise debilitated are often given glucose or dextrose in solution. This provides an immediate source of energy.)

FATS

Highly digestible fats provide essential fatty acids and about 2 $\frac{1}{4}$-times as much energy as an equal quantity of carbohydrate. It is easy to see why an egg yolk contains 33% fat versus only 1% carbohydrate: fat is by far the more energy-concentrated food. The growing chick will be assured of a plentiful energy supply which occupies the smallest space possible, as dictated by the limitations of the egg.

Fat deposits are laid down in an animal's body when there is excess fat (or excess carbohydrate) in the diet. These fat reserves are drawn from when the animal needs more energy than is supplied by the diet. Note that the nature and composition of body fat can vary considerably depending on the diet. This is a point to consider when raising animals for slaughter if the fat is also going to be used. Research will probably have to be done to establish what effects different diets will have on emu fat.

Fats improve the palatability of a feed ration as well as its general consistency.

PROTEINS

Since the animal body is made up mainly of protein, a good source of dietary protein is needed in all species, in particular during the period of **growth** (when the amount of body protein is actually being increased) and **reproduction** (when protein is needed by the female especially, to support the growth of an embryo or the laying of many eggs.) The "building blocks" of proteins are amino acids, and each species of animal /bird has a set of amino acids which are essential to it, i.e. must be provided in the diet.

This set of amino acids varies from species to species, and may even vary within the species for different stages of life, since a few more amino acids are often required for the growth process than for maintenance of the full-grown animal. This is part of the reason for having different "grower" diets, "maintenance" diets and "breeder" diets. As long as the essential amino acids and a sufficient source of protein are provided, other amino acids (non-essential) can be synthesized from these.

We do not know yet what the essential amino acids for emus are. However, based on the fact that adequate growth and egg production occur when emus are being fed diets which have poultry feed as their basis, we can assume that their amino acid needs are adequately met within these feeds. The balances may not necessarily be ideal, but are at least adequate. Protein or amino acid deficiencies in most species of breeder birds would generally cause a decline in egg production, without affecting hatchability.

Protein quality varies between different feed sources. Not all proteins are readily digestible, but this is unfortunately not reflected in the information given on feed bags. The digestibility of some proteins is improved by heat processing, while for other proteins, heating reduces quality. The key factor is to use reputable feed companies who have a knowledgeable nutritionist on their staff, and who pride themselves on using high quality raw materials.

While some livestock farmers give their breeder animals a "protein boost" by raising the protein level temporarily for two or three months just before the onset of production, the use of very high-protein feeds on a continuous basis is not only economically unfeasible but may also be detrimental to the long-term productive life of the animal. (See **Section 6.10**). It is interesting to note that the generally recommended protein levels for breeder chickens and turkeys, as set forth by the U.S. National Research Council (Washington,D.C.) are between 14% - 15%.

VITAMINS

These are generally classified into two groups: fat-soluble (Vitamins A,D,E and K) and water-soluble (the B-vitamins. Vitamin C is also water-soluble but is not a dietary essential for birds). The main difference between the two groups is that the fat-soluble vitamins can be stored in the body, whereas any excess in the daily intake of the water-soluble vitamins tends to be excreted. Not only does this mean that deficiencies in the B-vitamins will be the more common, but also that there is little chance of toxic effects due to overdosage. The fat-soluble vitamins, however, can be toxic in excessive amounts.

Vitamin A is necessary for proper reproductive function, and for maintaining a normal epithelium, notably in the eyes and nose. A vitamin-A-deficient diet in chickens will lower the bird's resistance to upper respiratory infections. Tear glands in the eye dry up which can lead to eye infections, characterized by the gumming-together of the eyelids. This condition has also been observed in emus, but it is not known whether it was as a direct result of Vitamin A deficiency. Vitamin A is stored in the liver.

Vitamin E is also necessary for normal reproduction. In poultry chicks, deficiency results in "encephalomalacia" or "crazy-chick disease" or sometimes, muscular dystrophy. A similar condition, where the head tucks under the body between the legs and the chick sometimes runs backwards, has been observed in young emu chicks. Injecting with Vitamin E and selenium usually helps, and some cases recover spontaneously, e.g. when the new chick starts to eat properly. Adding wheat germ oil, a rich source of Vitamin E, to the diet may hasten recovery once the chick is eating. (Note: Be careful with dosage of injectable Vit. E and selenium, since too much selenium can be very toxic.)

Vitamin D3 is important for the proper assimilation of calcium and phosphorus from the diet, as well as its deposition for normal bone growth. It is useful in preventing rickets and thin-shelled eggs. Some Vitamin D is obtained from the action of direct sunlight on the skin, but it is usually added to the diet as well. Note that the closing up of birds for long periods, e.g. due to inclement weather, means that a nutritional deficiency of Vitamin D may occur. Adding small quantities of cod-liver oil (a rich source of both Vitamin A and D3) to the feed may be beneficial in such cases.

Vitamin K is necessary for the normal clotting of blood.

The B-vitamins are necessary for many normal growth processes. Some deficiency symptoms have already been listed (**Section 6.4**). Other deficiency symptoms include dermatitis, poor feathering and slow growth. Vitamin B-12, which must be obtained from animal sources, is essential for chick growth. Most B-vitamins are also necessary for proper development and hatchability of eggs (since this is also a growth process). This is further discussed in **Section 10.8.**

MINERALS

The minerals and trace elements are necessary not only for normal skeletal growth but also for many other body functions. For instance, **sodium**, **potassium** and **chlorides** help maintain correct fluid balances in the body. **Iron** is needed for the formation of red blood cells, and in increased amounts during egg production (to satisfy the needs of the developing embryo).

Calcium and **phosphorus**, along with smaller quantities of **magnesium**, are needed for proper bone growth. Phosphorus also has an effect on fertility. The correct ratio of calcium to phosphorus in feeds is between 2:1 and 1:1, with calcium comprising no more than 2% of the diet. Note that many of the minerals and trace elements are antagonistic, i.e. they compete for absorption in the gut. This is why excessively high levels of any mineral can completely upset or inhibit the absorption of several others. Thus an excess in one results in a deficiency in others. Excess iron, for instance, can inhibit the absorption of phosphorus in the gut. This in turn may upset the calcium/phosphorus ratio to the extent that calcium is not well absorbed either, and in severe cases, skeletal deformities or "rickets" may result.

Fig. 6.2 - THE "BALANCED DIET"

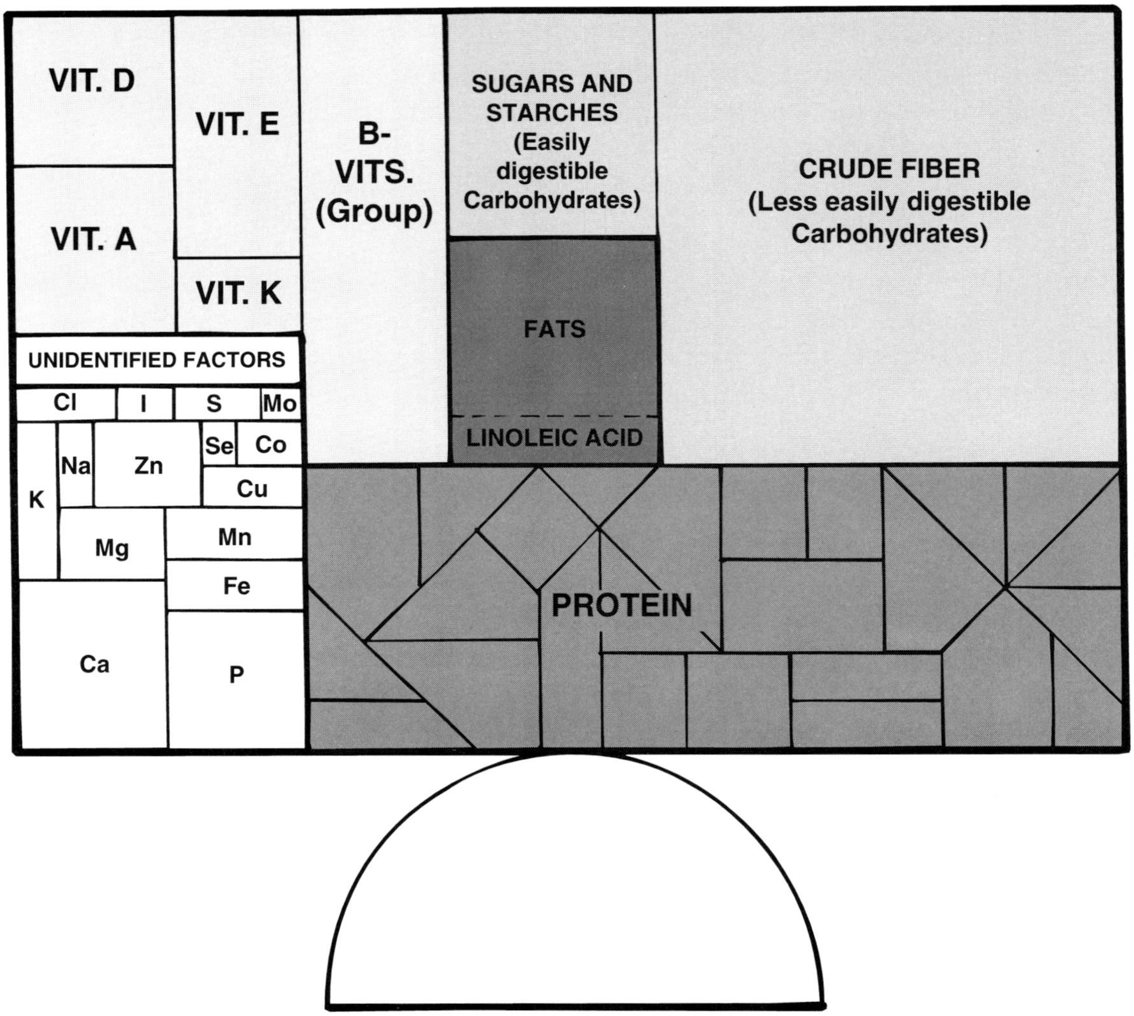

MINERALS (and unidentified factors)

VITAMINS (Fat-soluble and water-soluble)

CARBOHYDRATES (Including fiber as well as starches/sugars)

PROTEINS (The blocks represent different amino acids)

FATS (Including linoleic acid, an important essential fatty acid)

The roles of the trace elements **manganese** and **zinc** in preventing skeletal deformities have already been discussed (**Section 6.4**). In addition, manganese also has an effect on fertility. **Iodine** is needed for the manufacture of the hormone thyroxine in the thyroid gland, which in turn stimulates growth, sexual development and later, egg production in the hen. A symptom of deficiency in most animals is "goiter", an enlargement of the thyroid gland.

Iodine, as well as **copper**, **cobalt** and **selenium**, can be deficient in the soil in certain areas, and are therefore also deficient in the plants that grow there and in the feed made from these plants. A good feed manufacturer, therefore, should be well aware of any problems in his own area and make the necessary adjustments to the feed. Note that any elements required in trace amounts, e.g. selenium, can be TOXIC in higher amounts. For this reason, mineral and trace element supplementation in feeds is best done by the feed manufacturer. He should also have a good idea of what effect the addition of one substance will have on the others.The emphasis on balance in any good diet cannot be overstressed. While we do not as yet know all the nutrient requirements of emus or their proper ratios, it is wise to stay within certain bounds recommended for chickens and turkeys to start with and not to exceed any toxic levels, particularly in mineral nutrition.

After this brief discussion of the interrelationship of many nutrients, **Fig. 6.2** can be reviewed. With the sum total of the constituents of the diet (excluding water) being represented by the rectangle balancing on a curved block, one can picture an excess or a deficiency in any nutrient causing the block to tilt, as the diet becomes "unbalanced". The body of an animal is able to cope with short-term deficiencies and excesses provided they are not too extreme, so there is room for the rectangle representing the balanced diet to rock back and forth a little. However, an excess or deficiency that is great enough will cause the rectangle to tilt so far that it falls off the block. The diet is now not balanced, and problems in the growth, or reproduction, or general health of the animal will result.

6.6 ADDITIONAL DEFICIENCY SYMPTOMS SEEN IN EMUS

In addition to those already mentioned, there are a few other abnormalities seen in emus which may be a result of dietary deficiency:

- Turned-in or "rolled" toes, in young chicks
- Knock-knees, in older chicks
- Twisted neck, in older chicks
- Dome-shaped back, in older chicks and adult birds

Turned-in toes usually straighten out within a few weeks on an adequate diet. Adding dry yeast to the diet (for B-vitamins) may be beneficial. Knock-knees may be caused by too fast growth coupled with too little exercise and possibly, lack of

B-vitamins. Yeast supplementation in the diet for several weeks has sometimes proved helpful. A higher-fiber diet may also be useful in restricting growth somewhat (while not restricting essential nutrients). This can be accomplished by adding fresh greens to the diet (kale, cabbage etc.) or by supplementing the diet with alfalfa pellets or rabbit pellets which contain a lot of alfalfa.

Twisted neck is occasionally the result of an injury, but there are probably nutritional causes as well, as suggested in **Section 6.10**. Twisted neck can also be a symptom of disease, as outlined in **Section 14.6**, but the bird will be quite obviously sick and debilitated in these cases. The reason for dome-shaped back is not known, but fortunately not many cases are seen. Such birds often do not seem to be able to mate successfully owing to the physical limitation, but it would be inadvisable to breed with them anyway since the deformity could be hereditary.

6.7 THE EFFECT OF GENETICS

To what extent "genetics" actually affects a bird's susceptibility to deformities is a much debated subject. This is because GENETIC FACTORS, in true-life situations, cannot be separated from ENVIRONMENTAL FACTORS, such as stress, climate, conditions under which the bird is being raised, concentration of harmful organisms, and of course, nutrition.

"Poor genetics" are often blamed for deformities in chicks, simply because it is easier to cast the blame on something over which one has no control. A good emu farmer, however, should consider the possibility of a genetic problem only after he has exhausted all other possible causes. After all, there are some genetic differences in birds that are not really genetic problems. They simply need a change in management technique.

A good example of this is in the incubation of eggs, where all the eggs from one pair of birds die just before hatching. If the problem is found to be insufficient weight loss, the simple act of incubating all such eggs under drier conditions may produce a crop of beautiful, big, healthy chicks. If the farmer had decided the problem was "genetic" and had sold the birds, he might in fact have gotten rid of his genetically best pair of birds.

Similarly, on a "borderline deficient" diet, some chicks will develop leg deformities while others do not. This does not necessarily mean that these chicks are inferior and the parent birds should be culled from the breeding program. In fact, it is often the bigger chicks (with correspondingly larger weight gains as they grow, and perhaps faster growth rates) that develop the problems, in particular during "growth spurt" periods which occur several times during the first year. Some of the smaller chicks in a group may also develop the same problems on a "borderline" diet simply due to inadequate space at the feeders or too many chicks together, causing smaller birds to get crowded out and to consume less feed as a result. Other reasons for deformity in a chick could be inadequate breeder nutrition at the time the egg was being produced, or some other stress (e.g. infection) at that time.

The reason for some chicks and not others developing deformities on a "borderline" diet will usually be due to differences in metabolism, which **is** an inherited factor, causing some birds to need less of a certain nutrient than others, perhaps because they are slower-growing or assimilate the nutrient better. This is not a genetic problem, because on an adequate diet, all the birds would grow and develop normally. The birds that do not develop deformities are simply better adapted (genetically) to an inferior diet.

At this time, it is doubtful whether there are any widespread, serious genetic defects among emus around the U.S., since they really have not been farmed and "in-bred" for long enough. While some birds will tend to be larger, better-looking or more productive than others, these are genetic tendencies, not genetic problems. The tendency of most emu chicks, if they have been properly incubated, fed and cared for, is to remain very robust and healthy.

6.8 FOODS RICH IN VITAL NUTRIENTS

Deficiency diseases have been recognized for several hundred years, as has the fact that specific foods are helpful in their prevention and treatment. Old farmers' handbooks cite the following feedstuffs for the growth and maintenance of healthy poultry chicks:

- **Alfalfa meal** - provides Vit. E and A, B-vitamins, fiber, calcium, trace elements
- **Sour (curdled) milk, e.g. buttermilk, yogurt** - Calcium and phosphorus, Lactobacillus bacteria, protein, B-vitamins, trace elements
- **Yeast (baker's or brewer's)** - B-vitamins, protein, phosphorus, trace elements
- **Yellow corn** - Energy, Vit.A and some Vit.E
- **Chopped liver, bloodmeal** - Vit. B12, iron, phosphorus, Vit. A
- **Bonemeal** - Calcium, phosphorus
- **Cod-liver oil** - Vit. D3 and A.

The fact that farmers a few decades ago may not have known exactly what vitamins in these feeds helped prevent problems, did not make the feeds any less effective. These feedstuffs (among others) still form the basis of many poultry diets.

Because the B-vitamins (notably riboflavin, niacin, choline, pantothenic acid and B-12) are the most likely to be deficient in feed, owing to their more rapid deterioration, the addition of yeast, yogurt or alfalfa meal to emu chick diets has proved very helpful in the treatment and prevention of leg/foot deformities caused by B-vitamin deficiencies. Yogurt also provides Lactobacillus bacteria, which are the "friendly" bacteria needed in the gut to help prevent the growth of harmful bacteria, and to aid in digestion.

6.9 FACTORS INVOLVED IN PUTTING TOGETHER A GOOD EMU FEED

Because proper emu feeding trials have not at this time been conducted to any appreciable extent, the mixing of a proper diet for emus is still very much a matter of educated guesswork. Since this is the case, good feed manufacturers should try to be as educated in their guesswork as they possibly can. This calls for a good study of the bird itself, as outlined in previous sections, before starting to put figures on paper or ingredients into the feed cauldron.

- **Starter diet** - the main concern here would be to use a small pellet or large crumble, which the emu can easily see and pick up in its beak. Adequate vitamin supplementation (in particular of B vitamins), a good calcium-phosphorus and mineral ratio as outlined in **Section 6.5**, lower protein levels than poultry starter feeds but high energy levels, should be some of the goals to strive for.

- **Grower diet** - a larger pellet can now be used, with basically the same nutrient balances as in starter feed. If there seems to be a danger of excessive weight gain during this period, it may be a good idea to increase fiber content somewhat in the grower diet. It should be remembered that the first year is crucial to the continued good performance of the bird, and any damage done to the skeleton as it grows (because of nutritional deficiencies) can never be undone, once growth has stopped. Given the choice, it is better to have leaner chicks than fatter chicks. One can always "fatten up" lean chicks later, but one cannot undo skeletal damage caused by excessive weight gains, nor other problems related to early obesity such as a shortened reproductive life.

- **Breeder diet** - keeping in mind what an egg consists of, it is obvious that the diet of the hen must be fortified with the same constituents, since she has to produce hatchable eggs. Iron, fat, protein, plenty of B-vitamins, vitamins A,D,E, and K, manganese and calcium are all important egg constituents. As discussed in **Section 13.3,** in order not to cause problems in the male, the extra calcium should be given separately so that the male's system is not overburdened but the female can eat what she needs.

When minerals are added to feed, they are generally in the form of either sulfates, carbonates or oxides. The sulfates (e.g. manganese sulfate, copper sulfate) are the most soluble and the most available form of the nutrient to the animal. The least available forms are the oxides, although still available to some extent. Ferric oxide is the exception: it is totally indigestible and useless as a source of iron. Iron should be added in the form of ferrous sulfate. A look at the ingredients given on a feed tag should therefore give some sort of idea as to availability of mineral nutrients in the feed.

When no emu feeds are available, or none that have been sufficiently tested, emus can successfully be grown out on about a fifty-fifty mixture of 16%-protein rabbit pellets (the kind that contain at least half alfalfa) and 17% poultry lay pellets. Breeder birds have done well on the same mixture, but with more of the lay pellets and less of the rabbit or alfalfa pellets. A good vitamin/mineral supplement can be added if necessary, along with small quantities of corn chops two to three times a week for extra energy, especially during cold weather. Whole corn is not easily digested because of its tough outer coat, but cracked corn (corn chops) seem to be well utilized.

Corn chops should only be fed to growing birds in very limited quantities, since it tends to have a fattening effect in larger amounts. Alfalfa or rabbit pellets, however, are not fattening and can be safely given to young birds. Because alfalfa is so rich in B-vitamins and many other nutrients, it is unlikely that it would cause leg problems in growing birds. Besides, the birds seem to find the taste somewhat bitter, which limits the intake in many cases.

In any feed product made for emus, the use of high quality natural feed sources (such as yeast cultures for B-vitamins) is always a good idea. After all, there may still be some unidentified growth factors in feeds that have not yet been recognized, and over-purification could lead to their loss, resulting in an "unbalanced" diet.

Levels of FIBER in feeds used successfully on emus vary between 7 -15%, with ranges around 9-12% the most common.

6.10 THE DANGERS OF HIGH PROTEIN LEVELS IN EMU FEED

Feeds that contain very high levels of protein - 25% and over - have been known to cause problems in emus, in particular young, growing birds. Again, remembering that good nutrition is a question of balance, it is possible to avoid problems related to high protein levels by raising levels of vitamins, minerals and other important nutrients as well. The result is a very concentrated diet which may cause the bird to grow faster and mature earlier, but whose long-term and possibly harmful effects have not yet been studied.

Catfish food and some varieties of dog food are examples of these high-protein feeds that have been used for emus. While the birds appear to relish this food, this does not necessarily mean that it is good for them any more than a child's preference for candy over vegetables is the best nutritional choice for him. Animals may be self-regulating in the wild, but when raising them as domesticated livestock, one cannot assume they will do the same, for these reasons:

1. They are not being offered the same types of food that they have access to in the wild

2. They are not free to roam and seek out different types of food

3. Confinement generally means the birds get less exercise than what they do

in the wild, so energy needs will probably not be as great. At the same time, there will be a greater tendency to overeat or to over-consume the wrong types of food out of boredom or simply because it is there. Therefore when high-protein food is fed **free-choice**, any problem due to the high protein levels will be augmented because the feed is continually available. Over-consumption may also occur because of a deficiency which the birds are trying to compensate for by eating more. Finally, overeating may take place simply because the food tastes so good it is irresistible to the birds, though not necessarily healthy for them.

Potential problems with high-protein feeds designed for other animals

The high incidence of twisted necks, crooked backs, and knock-knees among young emus which have been fed exclusively on catfish food during their first year of life - particularly if fed free choice, with no supplements - may be due to at least 4 factors:

1. **Insufficient B-vitamins in diet**

The higher the protein level, the higher the levels of the B-vitamins in particular need to be, since these are the ones most directly involved in growth. Moreover, they cannot be stored in the body for long periods of time. In poultry and many other birds, deficiencies in different B-vitamins result in bone abnormalities, "slipping" of tendons and torticollis (twisted neck) to name a few. In the emu, anything that causes a twisted neck also has the potential of causing a crooked back, since the emu's thoracic vertebrae are not fused like those of a chicken and are therefore susceptible to being pulled out of alignment.

2. **Incorrect amino acid balance**

Every species of animal has a certain set of amino acids that are essential to it, and because of additional needs during GROWTH, the young animal may have a larger number of essential amino acids than the adult of the same species. Even species that are anatomically very similar may differ not only in their particular amino acid needs, but also in the proportions needed. While the protein in a particular commercial diet always supplies more than just the essential amino acids for that species, it is still unlikely that a diet designed for a fish, for instance, would have the ideal amino-acid balance for a running bird such as the emu. Amino acids, obtained from the digestion of the proteins in the diet, are used to build body proteins such as muscles, organs, tendons and nerves. Therefore, a serious imbalance or deficiency could easily result in corresponding abnormalities in the soft tissues of the body, e.g. poor or weak tendon growth which could result in tendons springing out of place due to the abnormal strain and causing crooked neck.

3. **Incorrect mineral balances**

A deficiency of the trace element MANGANESE will cause perosis or "splayed leg" in poultry and turkey chicks, and appears to do so in emus too. Lack of the correct amount of manganese, or excesses of other minerals which prevent the absorption of sufficient manganese, could conceivably cause both leg and neck problems.

4. **Low fiber**

Emus on high-protein, low-fiber (less than 5%) diets tend to consume more grass and other greenery in their pens, if it is available. A higher quantity of fiber than that found in catfish food/dog foods etc. may well be necessary for the proper functioning of the emu's digestive system, whether or not the emu can actually get much out of the fiber in terms of nutrients. (The same is true for humans, after all, who are not able to digest fiber to any extent.) Poor absorption of nutrients by the gut for any reason can bring about nutritional deficiencies, which in turn can cause deformities in neck/back/legs.

A very real danger in the continuous feeding of extremely high-protein feeds is the continual strain this puts on the kidneys to get rid of the toxic nitrogenous compounds that result. This extra burden may shorten the bird's productive life as well as its lifespan. While this may not matter much in birds raised for slaughter, it would definitely have a deleterious effect on breeder birds, since all the organs might "wear out" quicker.

Breeder birds also tend to become quite fat on catfish food or dog food, and obesity in any animal will lower production by making the animals sluggish and less interested in breeding, as well as less fertile and more prone to problems,such as egg-binding and egg yolk peritonitis in the hen (**Section 13.4 & 13.5**). Again, the raising of fat birds might not be a problem in birds being raised for slaughter, but might actually be an advantage in terms of oil production—as long as the quality of the meat or the fat itself was not compromised.

In general, the higher the protein level of a feed, the more it costs. If the protein level in a feed is much higher than what is actually needed, the farmer could actually be spending a lot of money enhancing the protein content of his birds' droppings. This is obviously not economically feasible. Some types of catfish food, when fed to emus, cause particularly odorous droppings which attract a tremendous amount of flies and other insects. Not only can these be bothersome to the emus (especially stinging insects) but they can also be carriers of disease.

In most practical rations fed to emus, a protein level of 15 - 20% has proved sufficient and well able to meet the needs of the growing and producing bird, provided other nutritional needs (vitamins, minerals, energy, fat, fiber) are also adequately met.

In birds with twisted necks who were under a year old (i.e. still growing), improvements were noted when:

1. the diet was changed from catfish food/dog food to poultry lay pellets and rabbit pellets, and

2. a good vitamin/mineral supplement was added to the diet, and

3. the birds' necks were stretched and massaged daily over a period of time.

6.11 FEEDING PRACTICES

There are two schools of thought at the moment on the feeding of emus:

1. Feeding "ad lib" or "free choice", which basically means that the birds have access to feed all the time. As soon as the level in the feed trough starts to go down, it is replenished with more, so that feeders are never empty. The idea is that the birds will eat what they need and thus never suffer any lack or deficiency, and the owner does not have to worry about whether or not his birds are getting enough food.

2. Feeding a set amount of feed (which may vary between different seasons and different age birds) at a set time or times every day. In order to follow this method successfully, one has to have an idea to start with of approximately how much a bird of a certain age needs to eat in order to maintain his optimum weight and good health; also, one needs to know the difference both by looking and feeling, what constitutes an (a) skinny (b) normal and (c) overweight bird, both in adults and in chicks.

Even though the second method does call for keener observation of the birds, such observation is certainly never a bad thing and should be part of every good emu farmer's practices anyhow. We recommend (and use) the second method because of a number of advantages:

(a) **Economics** - research in poultry has shown that feed is utilized and metabolized more efficiently by the bird when there are "rest" periods between mealtimes rather than feed being eaten continuously (as tends to be the case when it is continually available.) This means not only that "mealtime" birds get more out of their feed and therefore do not consume as much as "ad lib" birds, but also that money is saved in addition because there is less waste from throwing out feed that has simply gotten old in the feed trough. Finally, when a known amount is fed every day, it becomes easier to make financial projections as to what kind of feed bill one can expect in a year, and thus planning a budget also becomes easier.

(b) **Dietary benefits** - if birds never "get to the bottom" of their feed trough since the feed is being continually replaced, they may actually be getting an unbalanced ration as important minerals and other micro-nutrients slowly sift down to the bottom of the trough. (This may not be as much of a problem in pelleted feed as it is in mash or granules.) In humid areas, there is also the problem of rapidly-growing molds and bacteria which may start to grow in any feed that is allowed to sit for a while, and this can cause all sorts of intestinal problems in the birds. In the case of chicks, any feed placed directly under a heat lamp for a longer period can actually "cook away" some of the essential nutrients. In short, when the birds can "clean up" their feed every day, one can be sure that they are taking in the proper balance of nutrients. Also, the feed is always fresh.

(c) **Routine** - a set routine is beneficial for all animals, and helps to reduce stress. Feeding at a set time (or times) each day provides such a routine, and is also a good time to collect eggs during the laying season as the birds are usually too busy eating to even notice the eggs being picked up.

(d) **Taming-down** - no wild, stressed bird is a good producer. The presence of a human or humans on a regular daily basis, in connection with a good stimulus (feed) keeps the birds tame and used to human beings. Such birds experience less stress on handling or moving and settle down more easily in new surroundings. Having tame and docile birds also reduces the mortality/injury rate caused by terrified birds running into fences and damaging themselves.

(e) **Detection of illness** - one of the earliest signs of illness in most animals is going "off their feed". This may be difficult to tell when birds are fed free-choice. However, most "mealtime" birds are hungry enough by feeding time to go straight to the feeding trough to eat; if they do not, or if they suddenly start to leave a significant amount of feed uneaten, this is a good early warning signal that something may be wrong. All problems are more easily cured if caught in the early stages, and chances of recovery much better than having to deal with a bird whose illness has gone unnoticed for quite some time. (Note, however, that it is quite common for many emus to reduce their feed intake just prior to and during the breeding/ laying season. Moving to a new location may also cause birds to stop eating, sometimes for several days.)

(f) **Prevention of problems related to over-eating** - Finally, it must be remembered that any animal in confinement may tend to overeat if unlimited quantities of food are supplied, simply because there may be little else to do, or the feed ration happens to be particularly palatable. (Even humans do this, in spite of knowing better!) An overweight bird is not a healthy bird; in fact, fat adults are usually less productive than their leaner counterparts, and chicks that gain too much weight too quickly may develop leg problems. Fresh greens added to their diet is always beneficial for chicks. Alfalfa pellets can also be added to the diets of growing birds any time there is concern as to whether the birds are "getting enough". Since it is high in fiber and good nutrients but is not very palatable to most emus, there is little risk of over-eating, even when fed free-choice. Young birds will usually eat alfalfa pellets more readily than older emus.

The correct amount of feed per bird is a much discussed topic, and will depend a lot on the balance of nutrients in the feed itself as well as on the age and condition of the individual bird. When more research has been done on the balance of nutrients needed by emus of various ages, we will be able to settle more precisely on approximate quantities required as well. On a diet consisting of a balanced poultry lay pellet, periodically mixed with rabbit pellets (containing a lot of alfalfa) and cracked corn, 1 pound of feed per adult bird per day is a good MAINTE-

NANCE quantity of feed. If a bird has just finished laying season or is in poor condition for some other reason, then obviously the feed needs to be increased until the emu farmer is satisfied with the bird's condition. At this point he can return to the maintenance amount of feed.

6.12 USE OF BULK FEEDERS

While purchasing feed in bulk or mixing it in bulk may seem more economical at first than buying it bagged, caution should be exercised especially in humid or hot climates, for the following reasons:

- Overheating of feed may "cook away" some essential nutrients
- Dampness can cause growth of certain dangerous molds/fungi, notably Aspergillus
- Feed containers which are open at the top may attract vermin (rats, mice) which can contaminate the feed with their droppings
- Feed loses its freshness and gets old, less palatable and less nutritious

Some climates are definitely more suited to the use of bulk feeders - whether for storage or for feed dispersal to animals - than others. In hot humid climates, the losses experienced due to some of the problems listed above may make it more economical to buy bagged feed, and to feed on a daily basis. Many birds refuse to eat damp or stale feed.

6.13 OTHER FEEDING CONSIDERATIONS

Other than feed itself, birds must always be given access to plenty of fresh, clean WATER, as well as STONES/GRAVEL/GRIT of various sizes to utilize for grinding up feed in the gut. The different sizes are important for growing birds, as their needs may vary with growth. Oystershell should never be supplied as a source of calcium to growing birds. This is because although it is highly digestible, it contains NO phosphorus, and would therefore result in an excessive calcium/ phosphorus ratio if consumed in sufficient amounts. In addition, if little or no grit/stones are supplied, oystershell tends to be over-consumed since unlike insoluble grit/stones, it keeps dissolving in the gut and cannot be used to grind up food. This makes the imbalance even worse. If used at all, oystershell should only be fed to breeder females, since they have a different calcium metabolism which allows for a much greater calcium/ phosphorus ratio. Poultry hens are often given oystershell as a supplement. Like limestone or eggshell itself, it consists of calcium carbonate, but in a highly available form. Because hens have to mobilize so much calcium for the formation of eggshells, they appear to be able to tolerate much higher calcium/phosphorus ratios. One would assume the same to be true of emu females, although they have also been known to do quite well on normal calcium/phosphorus levels without extra calcium supplementation.

Some farmers feed crushed emu-eggshells to their breeder females, which the birds seem to relish, so there may well be an advantage in some form of calcium supplementation given free-choice.

If calcium supplementation is desired in young birds, it should be in the form of dicalcium phosphate (gray granules). This provides calcium and phosphorus in the proper ratios. Before supplementing with any nutrient, the amount already present in the feed should be considered. Over-supplementation with any one thing can disrupt the "balance" of a diet as discussed in **Section 6.5**.

Adequate space at feeders is another consideration in feeding large groups of young birds. A large number of "feeding stations" will help prevent overcrowding and will ensure that each bird gets a fair share of feed.

Dry, powdery feeds sometimes cause birds to "throw up" some of it, along with phlegm. Once moistened in this way, it is eaten with great relish by all the birds. "Throwing up" in this way is not a sign of sickness when birds appear healthy and normal in every other way, but it may be a sign that the feed needs to be mixed with something, perhaps a little oil or some greens, to moisten it.

"Greenery" i.e. some natural vegetation in the pens, while not a dietary essential, probably has some beneficial effects on the birds' digestive system as it adds some variety to the diet. Pecking at green stuff also helps keep the birds occupied and exercising. Adequate exercise is very important for good health and good growth of muscles and bones.

Birds are sometimes seen to peck at each other's droppings, and this does not appear harmful as long as there is no disease going around, and the birds have been wormed so they are free of intestinal parasites. It is even possible that the "recycling" of food that takes place in this way may be nutritionally beneficial, as the droppings have already gone through the digestive process once, and those nutrients still present may be more readily available the second time round.

6.14 MAKING CHANGES

If it becomes necessary to change the diet of young, growing birds, it should be done very slowly, with the new feed being gradually introduced. A vitamin/mineral supplement during this time is also not a bad idea, since any change necessitates an adjustment in the birds' metabolism. Deficiency symptoms (bent legs, enlarged hocks, stunted bone growth) have been seen in a group of birds that was phased down from a high-protein, vitamin-fortified diet to a lower-protein one. Birds of the same age that were on the lower-protein diet from the very beginning remained problem-free.

It is important to be CONSISTENT in the feeding of one's birds. If one jumps from diet to diet in order to follow the latest trend, and some deformities result, it may be impossible to figure out which diet or diets were the main cause of the problem.

Any good manufacturer of feed or feed supplement who claims his products will make birds bigger, better or more productive, must have evidence to back up such a claim. The emu farmer has every right to ask for details of any such research results. If none are available but the emu farmer still feels that the feed may be an improvement on his current feeding program, it would be wise to try the new feed on a small "control" group before putting all his birds on the new feed, especially if he is seeing adequate results on his current feeding program and simply wants to try to improve on it. By using a "control" group, not only can the differences in results be clearly seen between the current feed and the new feed, but also, if unforeseen problems are experienced on the new feed, at least the farmer will not have caused problems to his entire flock.

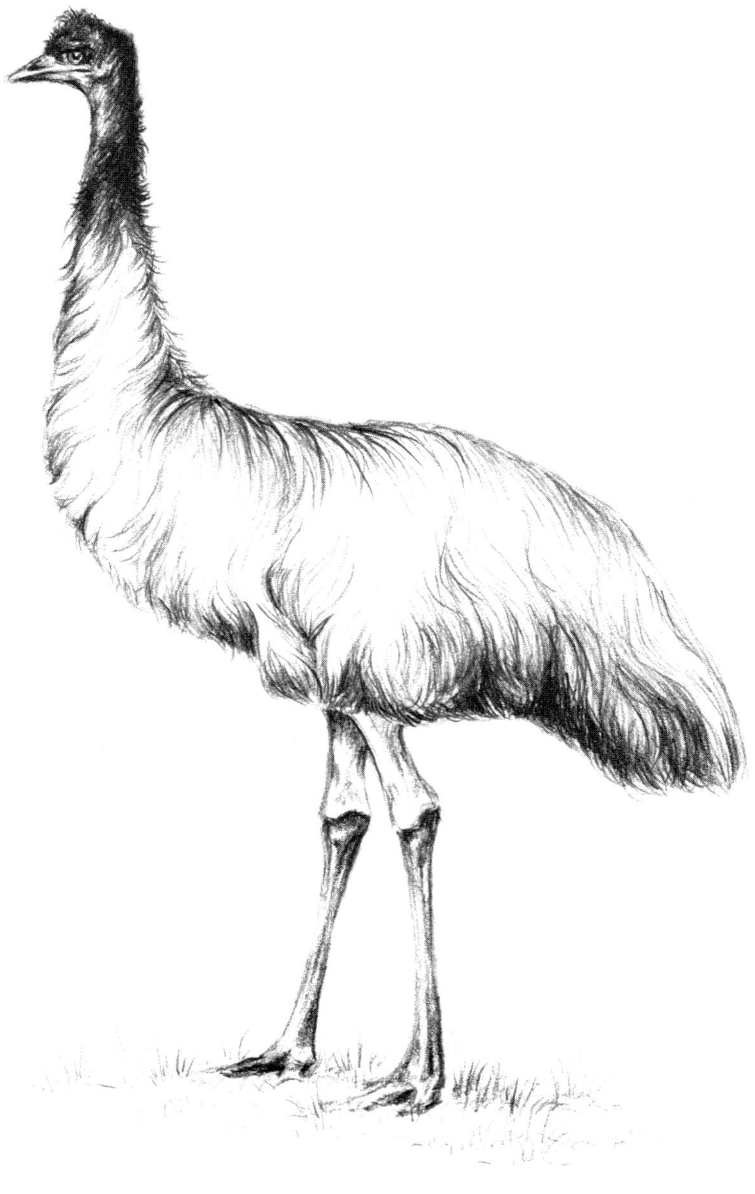

CHAPTER 7

The Breeding Season

Emus, like chickens or turkeys, make good farm animals because they are "indeterminate layers", i.e. they do not have a fixed number of eggs that they lay each breeding season. Instead, if an egg is removed (e.g. for artificial incubation) they will replace it. In this way, a larger number of eggs is generally produced under farming conditions than in the wild. Ensuring that both birds in a breeder pair are on a well-balanced diet also helps to ensure that the chicks that hatch will be healthy.

7.1 GENERAL FACTS

The emu breeding season takes place in the fall and winter. This means that in the southern hemisphere (Australia) it usually occurs between April and September, and in the northern hemisphere (U.S.) it runs from around October to March. The peak months are December, January and February.

Both the ratio of daylight hours to hours of darkness and the cooler temperatures probably have a stimulating effect on the complex hormone mechanisms that cause the birds to come into production. There are probably also other climatic factors that have an effect, such as extreme temperature fluctuations and high rainfall. The latter two have been reported to adversely affect laying in some birds, but more conclusive evidence is needed.

The age at which emus come into production varies with individual birds, and the level of nutrition from hatching up to that point also plays an important part. Poor nutrition (whether in the form of underfeeding, over-feeding or feeding an unbalanced diet) will generally cause a delay in the onset of production in most animals. Many emus breed and produce in their second year (as two-year-olds or coming two-year-olds), and most of those who do not, will be productive in their third year under good management conditions. The total number of productive years is not yet known, but emus in zoos have been known to still be producing chicks at age 16 years.

While some breeders have reported birds laying eggs when as young as 16 or 18 months, in particular on a very high-protein diet, it remains to be seen whether this is a lasting effect or simply one which will also cause the birds to "burn out" sooner. The subject of very high protein nutrition is discussed in **Section 6.10.**

At the onset of breeding season, behavioral changes will be noted in the birds. The male emu in particular becomes very friendly to anything he sees on two legs, including humans. His habit of following closely anyone who enters the breeding pen should not be mistaken for aggression; he is simply courting, and this can be confirmed by rubbing on his neck as he approaches. This stimulation will generally cause him to sit down in the breeding position. He may also attempt to peck, but this is also a display of affection as he will peck the back of the female's neck to encourage her to sit down for breeding, as well as during breeding itself.

Strutting about while displaying the neck feathers proudly is a sign both in males and females that they are getting ready for breeding season. In the female, the throat sac is sometimes seen hanging down as she makes drumming sounds. The male grunts a lot more than usual. These sounds are usually heard the most in the early morning and late evening, which is also when most mating seems to take place.

Once breeding season is in full swing and most of the mature birds are laying, there is generally very little fighting. Birds have been paired up (see **Section 7.2**) and most have settled in well and are very mellow. The females will usually lay an egg every 3 days, and breeding takes place in some pairs on a daily basis, in others less often. The breeding act itself is very simple and only takes about 30 seconds. The female raises her tail feathers, indicating that she is ready, and sits down, usually with tail feathers still raised. The male gets interested and may peck at her neck, back, and around the tail area. Then he squats on his haunches behind her, mounts while they are both in a sitting position, and mates with her for less than a minute while making grunting sounds. After this he gets up. There are no elaborate courtship displays as with ostriches and many other birds.

Some emu females take a break from egg-laying for a week or two in the middle of the breeding season, then resume with their regular cycle again. This is quite normal, and although such birds should be carefully watched in case they have in fact become "egg-bound" (see **Section 13.4**), one should not assume that just because they have stopped laying there is necessarily a problem. If the bird is eating and behaving normally, and no egg can be felt when her abdomen is gently palpated, there is probably no cause for alarm.

Three-sided shelters that are open to the outside so the birds can wander freely in and out at will are usually provided for breeder birds, particularly in wet areas or areas which experience freezing winter temperatures. Clean hay is provided in the shelters to encourage birds to nest there, and this ensures eggs will be laid in a clean, dry environment where they will be reasonably well protected against the elements. It is the practice of some farmers to put a blown-out "nest egg" in the shelter to encourage birds to start laying there. It is not known whether this does actually have any effect on stimulating egg-laying or on where to lay the egg, since one cannot know what the hen would have done, had the nest-egg not been there.

It is important to provide as stress-free an environment as possible to the breeder birds. Visitors should be kept to a minimum, and a regular feeding schedule is important. The birds generally cut back on their feed during breeding season, so the time to feed birds for breeding is actually before breeding season, since this is when they build up their reserves. Nevertheless, since the birds are eating less it becomes even more important to feed them right, and many emu farmers add a vitamin/mineral supplement to the birds' feed or water on a regular basis. Cracked corn may be provided periodically for extra energy, in particular when it is cold. It should not be fed in large quantities, however, as it may make the birds fat. Limestone or other extra source of calcium is usually provided free-choice in the breeder pens due to the female's high calcium requirements during egg production. This way, the female can consume what she needs, while not burdening the male's kidneys with excessive amounts of calcium. (See also **Section 13.3**).

Green stool, the color of emu eggs, is sometimes seen in breeder pens prior to the onset of lay. Some birds, however, will lay eggs through an entire season without any green coloration to the stool at all. The presence or absence of green stool is therefore not an accurate way of predicting whether or not a female emu is going to lay.

7.2 PAIRING UP POTENTIAL BREEDERS

Great care should be taken in this important part of emu farming. Many emu farmers with only a few young birds have no problem whatsoever in pairing them up. However, any farmer that has a large number of emus to pair up will encounter some aggressive birds. Aggression in emus is seldom directed at a human being, but usually at other emus, as attempts are made to establish dominance.

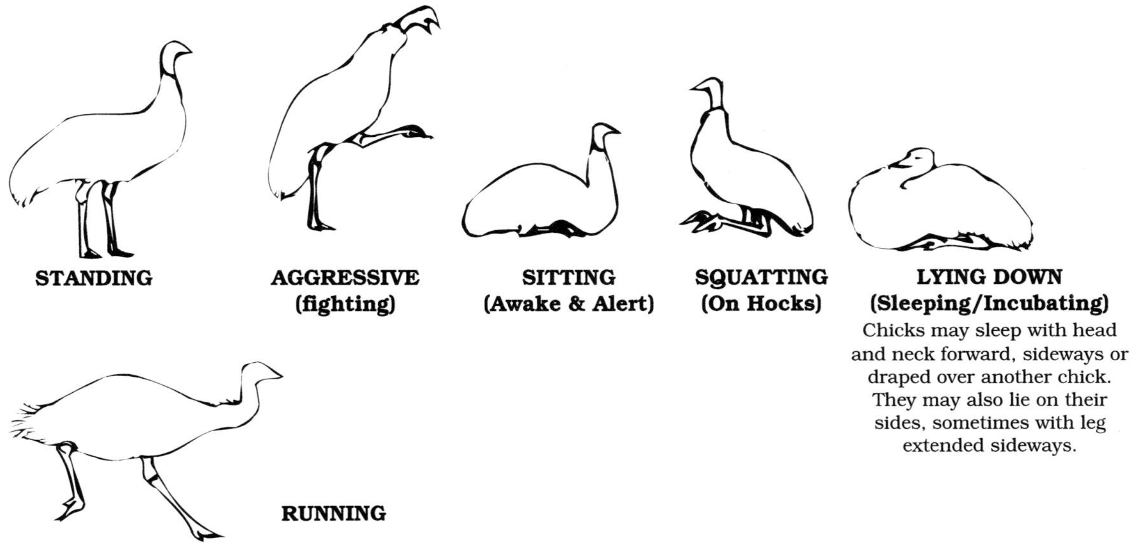

Fig. 7.1 - Some normal emu positions.

A second problem is the pairing up of birds that are not "compatible" - for some reason they simply are not interested in one another and will not produce fertile eggs together. While this situation is less dangerous than pairing up birds that fight, the economic end results are the same: no chick production.

Emus do very well if they are given the opportunity to choose their own mates. This may not be possible in every farming situation, but it does help in the pairing up of birds, particularly young potential breeders. When birds are seen together very often and especially if they sleep close together at night, chances are that they will team up successfully. The time of year is important, however. Since the most fighting/chasing among emus seems to occur from mid- to late summer, peaking in the hot months of July and August, birds should not be regarded as "paired up" until after this time has passed. Hormonal changes in the birds during this time, as they approach sexual maturity, may cause behavioral changes to the extent that a bird may make every effort to chase another out of its pen, with whom he got along quite well before. Most emu farmers therefore wait until fall (September onwards) before they start pairing up their birds.

A good way to get one's emus teamed up is to put single females in the breeder pens while leaving the males in the alley. (This is another good reason to design one's pens with an alley or walkway between them.) Generally, a group of females will tend to do more fighting amongst themselves than a group of males, so by splitting up the females and letting the males remain in a group, this problem is avoided. As breeding season approaches, most males have only one thing on their minds: courting anything on two legs. The birds can be checked nightly to see which males are starting to stay around which females, as well as if the females are responding by staying at the fence near "their" male. A lot of strutting, drumming and grunting occurs at this time, especially in the evenings. When a male and female have been observed together for 3 - 4 days in a row, they may be put in the same pen, keeping them under careful observation for several days in case either bird changes its mind and wants to fight. Injuries to birds are almost sure to result if they are in small breeder type pens and start to fight in earnest. Injuries may occur either from each other (kicking/lacerations) or from running into fences, trying to escape the attacker. Birds must be separated immediately if serious fighting begins. A couple of long-handled brooms may be helpful for separating birds without getting in the way oneself. A bird in trouble will, however, often spot an open gate immediately and head for it, so a person just needs to be there to close it quickly and contain the troublemaker in the pen.

Often a pair or two remain that just will not team up, and at this point there are just a few stronger measures to try which will sometimes work. Put these remaining birds into a larger pen - at least 50' x 100' or so - which ideally contains some brush and small trees to provide "cover" for any bird that is being chased, so that he can get away - and leave them until some type of pairing up starts to occur. If one bird continually chases the others, giving them no chance to settle down, she/he may need to be separated for a while. Some fighting may be due to frustration because one bird is ready to breed and another is not. Do keep birds separated as long as they are showing strong tendencies to fight, but remember that as the season progresses, most emus become more mellow. As young birds continue to mature sexually during the breeding season, a female may quite readily accept a male that she was trying to kill the week before. Patience and continuous observation are the key to successful pairing of young breeders.

A second method of pairing birds that tend to fight or show no interest in each other is to close them up in a dark stall or dark trailer. The birds are fed and watered in the darkness for about a week. They will not normally fight in a darkened area like this (although there have been some exceptions, and of course as with any change, the birds should be carefully monitored for the first day or two). Some birds will resume fighting once they are released, but more often they are happy to be out, have forgotten their problems and may even have bonded and be ready to breed.

A third and more widely used method of pairing birds is to split the breeder pen in half with cattle panels or other temporary fencing, and feed and water the birds at the fence that separates them. This gets the birds used to eating together without giving them the opportunity to fight, nor to simply ignore each other (since if one does not feed with the other, he may find his share eaten by his future mate. He will be hungry enough to make sure he eats with her by the next feeding time.) Once the birds start to sleep near the fence close to each other, the panel can be removed and the birds reintroduced. One should not ever be in a hurry to put young birds together, especially if they have a history of fighting. Waiting 2 to 4 weeks after seeing some positive results before actually pairing up the birds can only make the bonding better. Too often people want to speed things up because they hope the birds will lay sooner, and if one bird is still not quite ready, fighting may resume and you have to start from the beginning again.

Once a pair of emus has bred and produced fertile eggs with good chicks together for a season, that pair is usually kept together for the sake of convenience. They will usually continue to produce well year after year, so there is no reason to separate them or change mates. However, if one of the birds should die or if the birds begin to fight for some reason, the introduction of a new mate can be effected by one of the means already listed. Every emu can bond with a new mate: it may take some time and patience, but it should be noted that according to most sources, emus in the wild do not bond for life but only for a season, and sometimes less.

Apparently, an emu female in the wild often goes and lays a second clutch of eggs for a different male, once her own mate has begun to incubate (and therefore, has lost interest in breeding her). Some Australian emu farms which use male emus rather than artificial incubators to hatch their eggs, make use of this practice in order to get a better yield from their females.

It is not uncommon for an older breeder pair to skip a breeding season altogether after a few excellent years. The reasons for this are not yet known. A stress factor such as moving the birds to a new location may play a part, but since most emus do not seem to object at all to being moved, and some continue to breed and lay even if moved in the middle of breeding season, we might assume that the occasional skipped breeding season might just be Nature's way of allowing the birds to rest and catch up. After all, their total productive life is a very long one, and by continually removing eggs for incubation, we also cause the hen to lay more eggs per season than normal. Perhaps as more research is done to improve nutrition and genetics, less and less of this problem will occur. While the introduction of new mates may be attempted with an older breeder pair that is showing no interest in mating, it should be remembered that older birds will often resist change, and may give a new mate a severe beating. On the other hand, some young males which have reached sexual maturity very recently seem to be particularly virile, and an older female may sit down and allow a young male to breed her soon after they are introduced. If they continue to get along well they may be kept together for the duration of the season. If, after breeding, she starts to chase him around, he should be removed and the older male be put back in with his female. Sometimes the removal of the male and his subsequent re-introduction stimulates the pair to get on with breeding from that time on. If the old male continues to show no interest but it is obvious that the female is ready to breed, the male can again be removed and replaced with the younger, more virile male for as long as it takes him to breed the female. In effect, the younger male is acting as a "teaser" male which may help the female to get into the breeding and laying mode; this in turn may stimulate her own old male. While this may not be economically feasible once the emu enters the commercial market phase (because of the extra time and labor involved) it is certainly worth trying if time and opportunity allows. It can also work when a female is laying infertile eggs, i.e. her own male is not breeding her.

Note that an older breeder pair that has skipped a season need not be permanently separated or re-paired; often they will produce well together the following year.

What happens when a bird shows no interest at all in his/her own mate, but constantly paces the fence together with the bird next door? If the feeling appears to be mutual, swapping the birds around may be attempted.

Again, there is no hard and fast rule: it must be remembered that these birds are animals, not machines, and sometimes do not behave as we would expect them to. Only by doing as much "bird-watching" as possible, and by learning from what we observe, can we become successful emu farmers.

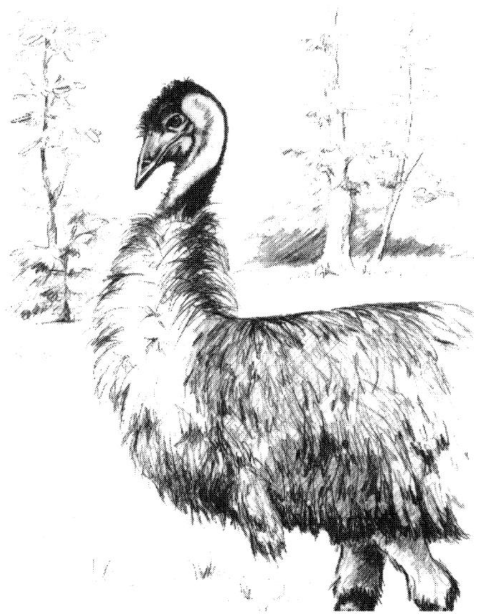

Strutting Emu

CHAPTER 8

The Path of the Egg

If emu farming was always as straightforward as picking up eggs, incubating them and watching them hatch into healthy chicks, there would be no need for this chapter. Unfortunately, problems do sometimes crop up. In order to solve these problems and come as close as possible to the ideal of successfully hatching as many eggs as possible it is necessary to understand as much as we possibly can about the whole process: from egg development in the hen to the growth of the embryo inside the egg into a chick.

8.1 THE BEGINNING

Unlike most mammals which have two functioning ovaries, most birds have only one. Generally, the left ovary is the one that develops, while the right remains rudimentary. This ovary contains thousands of follicles which have the potential of developing into eggs. When a bird is sexually mature and ready to produce eggs, its ovary resembles a cluster of grapes, all different sizes according to their stage of development.

The journey of an egg or "ovum" begins when it is released from the follicle which has encapsulated it up to this point, and drops into the funnel of the oviduct. The egg's path may easily be traced by following **Fig. 8.1**, as outlined in the next section.

8.2 REPRODUCTIVE TRACT OF THE EMU HEN

1. **Ovary** - Cluster of eggs or "ova" in various stages of development, located near the top of the back.

2. **Infundibulum** - "Funnel" of oviduct, into which the mature ovum drops when it is released from its follicle. This is also where fertilization takes place, if the bird has mated and there are sperm present.

3. **Magnum** - This is the area of the oviduct where layers of albumen ("egg white") are secreted onto the ovum. Note that the ovum itself is basically an egg yolk. The egg white, shell membranes and finally the shell are secreted onto the yolk as it moves on down the oviduct. Whether the ovum has been fertilized or not, the same process will occur, usually within the same time frame. Thus when an egg is first laid, there is no way of telling whether or not it has been

fertilized: a fertile and an infertile egg will look just the same.

4. **Isthmus** - In this portion of the oviduct, the shell membranes are secreted. These membranes are white, and there is an inner shell membrane which covers the egg contents (later, the developing chick) as well as an outer shell membrane which lies against the shell once the shell has been secreted. Between these two membranes, usually at the large end of the egg, the air space of the egg will form.

5. **Uterus** (Shell Gland) - The egg will spend the greatest amount of time in the uterus or "shell gland" - this is where the layers of hard shell are secreted onto the egg. In the emu, three distinctly colored layers will form the egg shell: an inner white layer, followed by a light green or aqua-colored layer, followed by the dark green outer layer. The light green layer is usually the thickest, the dark green the thinnest, like a "skin" over the egg. **Fig. 8.1** shows the uterus with an egg in it.

6. **Vagina** - This is the short passage between uterus and cloaca, through which the egg must pass in order to be laid.

7. **Cloaca** - Although not strictly a part of the reproductive tract, the oviduct culminates in the cloaca. The gut and the ureters also pass their (waste) products into this common chamber, before elimination occurs via the vent. Since the egg also has to be laid via the vent, one might wonder how the egg avoids becoming contaminated with feces on its way out. Some protection is no doubt afforded by the cuticle, a slimy transparent final secretion which gives the egg a slight luster when it has dried, but it is quite probable that the female everts the lower part of her oviduct to lay the egg in much the same way as during mating, so that the egg actually never comes into contact with any feces present in the cloaca. On occasion, there might be a white smear of uric acid on the egg, but this has never in our experience made any difference to the successful incubation of an egg. (Uric acid is the semi-solid white waste product produced by the bird's kidneys, the equivalent to urine, which is liquid, in mammals).

An egg may of course be laid in feces which is already on the ground, but contamination will rarely occur inside the bird.

The walls of the entire oviduct are extremely elastic, with many folds to allow for expansion and contraction as each egg moves on down. The eggs of a young bird in her first year of lay may occasionally have a blood smear or two on them. This is usually nothing to worry about as long as the problem does not continue or become worse. A lack of sufficient lubrication in some part of the oviduct, or slight "over-stretching" of the oviduct may have occurred, causing a small amount of bleeding which usually corrects itself. One should remember that a young bird's oviduct is not going to be as wide or as elastic as that of an older bird, which has already laid many eggs. It will stretch out a little more and become more flexible with time. Similarly, if a very large egg is laid, some blood may be found on it for the same reason.

Fig 8.1 - Reproductive tract of the emu hen.

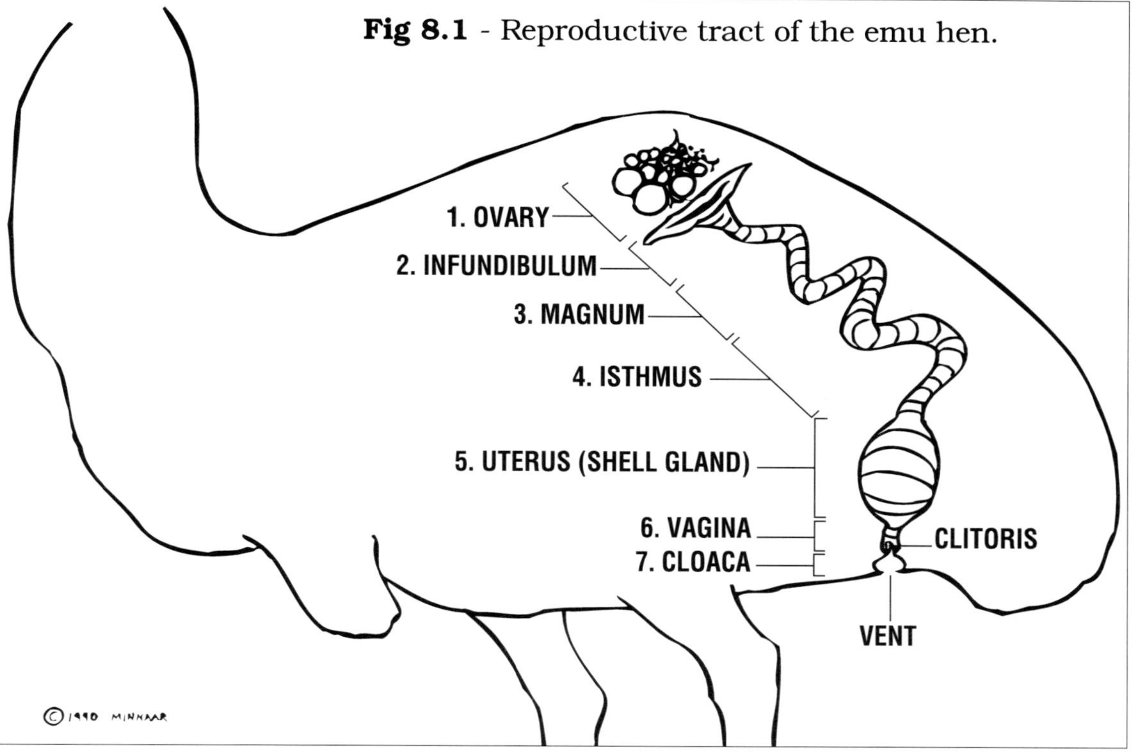

Some emu hens will pass a bright green stool (egg shell color) before laying their first egg. Unfortunately, this is not a good indicator of when the bird will actually start to lay since it can happen several days before the first egg, or several weeks. Most birds will lay sometime during the season if green stool has been observed on one or more occasions, but there will be a few exceptions. The green "stool" is probably due to excess secretions from the bird's uterus as it prepares for secreting green shell on the eggs. The green coloration is not necessarily an indication that there is already an egg in the oviduct.

Other unusual "stools" may also be seen in the birds' pen at this time - slimy transparent stools, yellowish-flecked stools, even stools with a little blood in them. If the female looks healthy and is eating and drinking, one can assume that these are simply extra secretions from the oviduct as it prepares to receive eggs. However, if there is an excessive amount of secretion or it continues for a long period, or the bird becomes listless, a veterinarian should be contacted. The bird may have an infection or be egg-bound (see **Section 13.4**) and will then require treatment and/or antibiotics. Blood in a stool or secretion should always be a cause for concern and extra surveillance.

8.3 THE EGG'S JOURNEY

Part 1. Down the Oviduct

The average emu female lays an egg every three days during the laying season. Some may be more irregular, producing an egg only every four, five or six days, but 3 days (72 hours) is the usual time period between eggs. Mature breeder females often get into the habit of laying their egg at a certain time of day as well, which makes it easy for the farmer to collect the eggs while fresh. Late evening is the most common egg-laying time, although some birds lay in the early morning and there will always be the exceptions who lay at any time of day.

Every species of bird has its own time-frame for the laying of eggs, and this does not necessarily correspond with the size of the bird. For instance, a chicken lays an egg every day; an ostrich, every second day; but an emu, which is smaller than an ostrich, lays every three days.

We can only guess at how long an emu egg spends in each portion of the oviduct. Since extensive studies have been done on chickens, however, and since the egg of any bird has to receive the same basic coatings, the table below illustrates how long an emu egg might spend in each section, by multiplying the known time periods for chickens by three.

Table 8.1 - *Possible time periods spent by emu egg in different portions of oviduct, in comparison with chicken egg.*

	CHICKEN	EMU
Infundibulum	¼ hour	¾ hour
Magnum	3 hours	9 hours
Isthmus	1¼ hour	3¾ hours
Uterus	20 hours	60 hours
TOTAL TIME:	24½ hours	73½ hours

Note that the chicken egg spends about 20 of its total 24 hours in the shell gland. This means that the emu egg could spend as much as 60 hours in its shell gland. If this is true, this would definitely be something to take into account before deciding that a bird must be "egg-bound" and taking drastic measures to "help" the bird lay the egg. Quite possibly an experienced person would be able to feel the egg in the uterus by palpating, long before that egg is actually ready to be laid. However, if it has been possible to feel the egg by palpating for a longer period than 60 hours, it is probably time to intervene (see **Section 13.4** on The Egg-Bound Hen). There should only be one egg in the oviduct at a time. In a normal cycle, after one egg has been laid the next yolk will drop into the oviduct.

Part 2. From Lay to Incubation: The Dormant Period

It is rare to see an emu egg being laid since it happens so quickly, and more often in the hours of darkness. However, a person who has the good fortune to observe this might see the hen squatting on her haunches rather than laying down completely, and then giving a slight push which hunches her body somewhat, whereupon the egg is dropped with a thump to the ground. This does not usually hurt it, unless dropped onto a sharp stone which may puncture the egg and render it useless for incubation. The egg will be shiny and wet, and will feel slimy to the touch if collected immediately. It is probably better to wait a few minutes and let this slimy layer (the cuticle) dry on the egg, before collecting it, since this dried cuticle provides a barrier against infection.

Once laid, the egg immediately begins to cool, as it has just left the warmth of the hen's body. The cooling will contract the egg contents somewhat, and the air space will begin to form between the inner and outer shell membranes. The cuticle dries onto the egg and "seals" it against bacteria, and the embryo goes dormant and will remain so, under the right temperature conditions, until the egg is incubated. The egg may be safely stored in the horizontal position for a period of 2 to 3 days at temperatures between 40°F and 60°F (4.5°C to 15.5°C) with 55°F (13°C) being considered the ideal storage temperature. It is quite possible that emu eggs could be stored a lot longer than this without harming the embryo, but more studies need to be done on this. Eggs in storage are usually turned twice daily by hand. While chicken eggs and other smaller or thinner-shelled eggs need to be stored in an area with higher humidity to prevent excessive weight loss (by evaporation) prior to incubation, this is usually not necessary with emu eggs, whose weight loss during storage tends to be negligible. Note that if storage temperature rises above 70°F, the embryo may start to develop but at an abnormally slow rate which will be harmful or fatal. Temperatures below 40°F over any length of time will also kill the embryo. An egg that has frozen solid is of no use for incubation; therefore, during freezing temperatures (32°F or below) eggs should be collected as promptly as possible. Some studies have attempted to show that storage of an egg prior to incubation will actually increase hatchability. In our experience there has been no difference in hatchability between eggs stored for a period prior to incubation and eggs incubated when freshly laid.

Note also that storage can never improve egg fertility, since an egg is either fertilized or not fertilized while it is still in the hen. By the time it is laid, if it was not fertilized there is no process known as yet that can make it into anything but an infertile egg.

It is interesting to note that in the wild the male emu does "store" some of his eggs too, before beginning to incubate them. The reason for this in Nature is of course that since the emu hen will only lay an egg about every three days, it will take around three weeks to lay a full clutch of eight or nine eggs. A synchronized hatch (all eggs hatching at roughly the same time) is important in the wild for better survival of the species, so it is understandable that the male does not begin to incubate immediately. Instead, he covers the eggs with leaves, twigs, dry grass or whatever happens to be available, in order to insulate them. When enough eggs have been laid and the male does begin to incubate, he usually goes into a trance-like state and loses interest in eating, breeding and just about everything else. This is apparently the point at which the female may go and find herself another male for whom she will lay a second clutch, if she is in a good state of nutrition and the breeding season is not too far along.

Part 3. The Incubation Period

Whether an emu egg is incubated naturally or artificially, it needs the following things:

1. Correct **temperature**, without too many extreme or lengthy fluctuations
2. Regular **turning**, to prevent the heavy yolk sinking and sticking to the bottom of the egg, or the embryo from floating upwards and sticking to the top.
3. Enough **air flow** to provide adequate amounts of oxygen to the developing embryos in the eggs and to help provide sufficient weight loss.
4. Correct **humidity** levels to promote optimum weight loss in the egg - not too high, nor too low.
5. An **infection-free** environment to prevent possible invasion of the egg by harmful organisms.

Gentle handling and correct positioning are also important.

If all these requirements are met and if the egg was fertilized, is not infected and contains all the nutritional elements that it should, then at the end of the incubation period the egg should hatch out into a healthy normal emu chick. The process of incubation is covered in detail in the chapter on Incubation and Hatching.

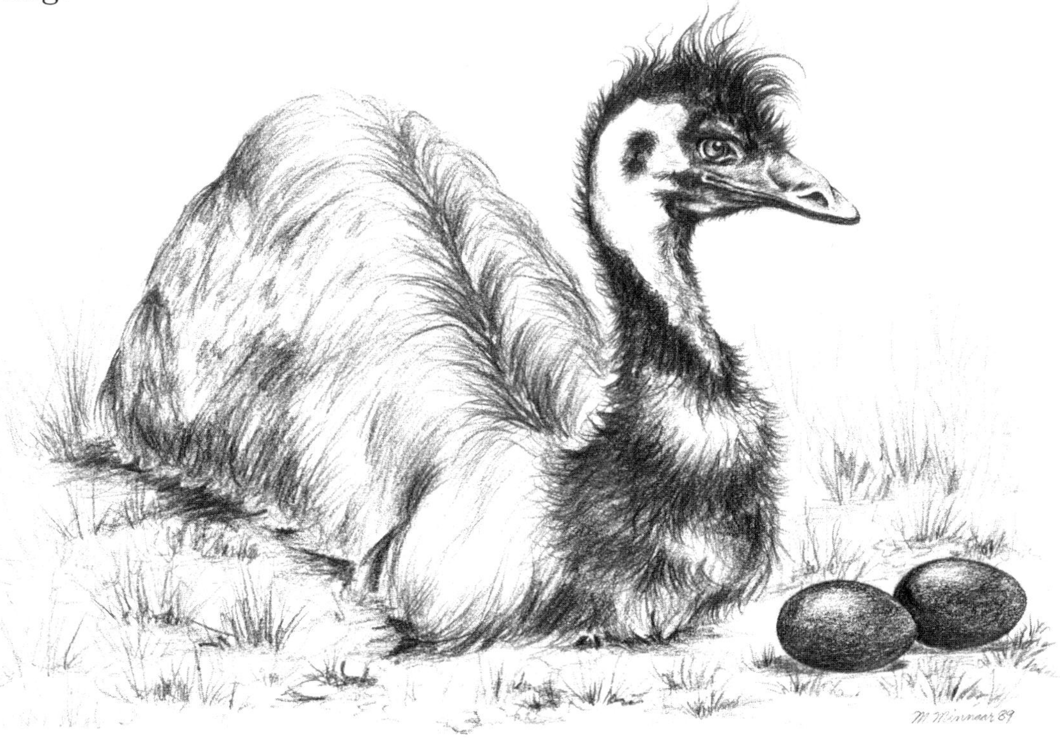

CHAPTER 9

Care of Eggs, Pre-Incubation

9.1 EGG HANDLING AND COLLECTING

Next to proper nutrition of breeder birds, the most important factor affecting hatchability of emu eggs is to start with a clean, dry egg. Eggs that are laid in the rain or mud are at much greater risk of infection and generally have very poor hatchability.

In order to lay clean, dry eggs the breeder birds must of course have a clean, dry place to lay them. In drier areas which do not experience freezing temperatures or much rainfall during winter, eggs laid outside on the ground can often be successfully incubated. However, in colder/wetter climates it will be necessary to provide the breeders with a shelter large enough for them to lie in comfortably. Placing bedding material such as hay or straw in the shelter will encourage the birds to use the shelter during cold nights and also, hopefully, to lay their eggs in it, since the hay provides nesting material with which the male can cover the eggs. The hay is replaced periodically to ensure it stays reasonably clean.

Eggs are usually laid either in the late evening or early morning, and most birds will settle into a steady routine of laying at roughly the same time of day every three or four days. In the beginning and at the end of laying season the cycle may be more irregular, and young first-time layers also tend to be more irregular to begin with. Once the birds have settled into a steady three-or four-day pattern, it is easy to anticipate when the egg is due and it can be collected soon after being laid. Collecting eggs while still fresh is the ideal.

Most birds will not object to their eggs being collected, as they generally become very tame and docile during breeding season. In order to cause the least amount of stress, it is a good idea to collect eggs during feeding time, if eggs are collected in the morning. This way the birds will be too busy eating to notice. If eggs are collected at night, it is best to move quietly around the birds and not use the flashlight any more than is necessary. As the breeding season continues, the male may be found already sitting on the fresh egg. He can then be gently lifted by grasping one of the legs tucked under him, and the egg can be removed. Usually the male is already in his trance-like incubation state, and will not offer any resistance to being lifted and put down again. It is as well not to leave the male any eggs to incubate himself (unless one wishes to do so at the very end of breeding season) since he will most likely stop breeding the female in order to devote himself fully to incubating his egg or eggs.

While some emu farmers take careful precautions to pick up eggs only with rubber gloves, and wash the eggs carefully prior to incubation, most of this is not necessary. Hands should always be clean prior to handling eggs, of course, but the egg itself has many natural barriers against infection since the ground on which it is laid in the wild (or the nest-hay on the farm) is by no means sterile. Indeed, by washing an egg prior to incubation, some of the egg's natural defenses may be removed.

Eggs should be collected into a clean container, and can either be marked right away or when brought inside for incubation. A clean towel, paper towels, or clean hay can be placed in the container to ensure the eggs do not roll around too much. Eggs are marked (numbered and dated) with a white colored pencil, marker or typewriter correction fluid. The type of marker used has never in our experience caused any detrimental effects to the developing chick. Stick-on tags are used by some farmers, but have the disadvantage of falling off at some stage during incubation, leaving you with eggs whose hatch date can only be guessed at. (This is another situation where egg-tapping proves very useful - see **Section 10.4**).

The farmer soon becomes very familiar with the eggs laid by different birds, to the extent that he can take the eggs laid by seven or eight different birds, lay them on the counter and know exactly which hen laid which egg. This is because each hen tends to lay eggs that are very similar to one another both in shape, texture, color and size. The only exception to this are first-time layers whose first few eggs are sometimes significantly smaller than subsequent eggs. As the oviduct stretches to what will become her "normal" width, the egg sizes become more uniform. Some of the many different varieties of eggs laid by emus are outlined in **Section 9.3**.

9.2 EGG HYGIENE

The egg is naturally equipped with barriers against invasion by harmful bacteria, and if laid under reasonably clean, dry conditions, it can be incubated without any further treatments. This is the ideal situation. A little sand or dry dirt on the egg is usually brushed off with a soft dry brush or paper towel prior to incubation.

Remembering that the transparent cuticle (final coating) has dried on the egg to effectively seal it against entry of harmful bacteria, it is probably better not to disturb this by wiping or rubbing with any wet cloths.

Eggs that are muddy or wet, however, may need some type of cleaning procedure prior to being incubated. In commercial poultry hatcheries such eggs would often be discarded rather than spending extra time and effort cleaning them and still running a risk that they might already have become infected. In emu egg incubation, however, we are still at a stage where all eggs with a chance of hatching are incubated. Some commonly used cleaning procedures are outlined below.

1. **Misting** - If eggs are dry but have some patches of caked-in dirt that cannot be removed by dry-brushing, some farmers will mist these eggs with a solution of disinfectant safe for eggs just before putting them in the incubator. The eggs then dry very rapidly in the incubator as the warm air blows on them. The idea behind misting is to kill any bacteria that still remain on the surface of the eggshell and thus prevent any contamination to other eggs. Misting will not kill any bacteria that have already entered the egg. Some people also mist periodically inside the incubator for much the same reason - to kill any airborne bacteria that may have been introduced. Misting is usually done very lightly - just a few squirts with the spray-bottle at a time - so as not to drastically alter the humidity in the incubator.

2. **Washing eggs** - If there is so much mud/dirt on the eggs that they need to be washed, they should be washed in a disinfectant solution which is at least 10°F warmer than the temperature of the egg. Disinfectants commonly used are solutions of Nolvasan, (chlorhexidine), Betadine or 1 - 2 tablespoons chlorine bleach per gallon of water. The egg can safely be completely immersed in such a solution for up to a minute, while gently washing off the dirt by hand. Pat dry with clean paper towels - do not rub hard, as the idea is to still leave as much of the protective cuticle on the egg as possible. The presence of the cuticle on the egg will make it feel slimy to the touch when immersed in water. The egg should be incubated as soon after washing as possible. Again, this only kills surface bacteria. The reason for the warmer water is to cause egg contents to expand, rather than contract to draw water in. Air bubbles are seen to escape from the pores, hopefully taking any bacteria with them.

3. **Antibiotic egg dipping** - Although not much work has been done with this method as yet on emu eggs, antibiotic egg dipping is the one cleaning process that can help destroy bacteria inside the egg. Its effectiveness may be less in emu eggs than in poultry or turkey eggs due to the greater thickness of the shell and differences in pores. Some good results have been reported with the dipping of ostrich eggs, however.

If fresh, the egg is first pre-warmed in an incubator for several hours, then immersed in the cold antibiotic solution (e.g. Tylosin) for 15 - 30 minutes. This should cause the egg contents to contract, drawing antibiotic solution in through the pores. The egg is then incubated. Weighing before and after dipping will show how much solution was actually taken in. This is the only situation in which an egg will gain weight, although by a very small amount.

Eggs that could benefit from antibiotic egg dipping would be those which were heavily contaminated e.g. with feces on being laid, and/or stayed wet and dirty for a long time before being collected. Also, eggs that have been contaminated in the incubator with the contents of a rotten egg which oozed or exploded might benefit. There could be a risk to the developing embryo, however, in immersing and cooling the egg for so long in the solution, especially one that has already started the incubation process. In addition, more work would need to be done on proper concentrations, the most effective soluble antibiotics and how often the treatment would need to be repeated.

9.3 INDIVIDUAL VARIATIONS BETWEEN EGGS

The type of egg most people come into contact with in their daily lives is the chicken egg, neatly packed with eleven others of almost identical shape, color and size in a box in the grocery store. We tend to forget that these eggs have already been pre-sorted and any weird shapes and extreme sizes have already been discarded. Thus, we are sometimes surprised at the variety of shapes, sizes, colors and textures among emu eggs, whereas in actual fact such differences do exist within most bird species. This section will deal with some of the different types of emu eggs one is likely to encounter during the course of a season.

1. **The Tiny Egg** - Usually, first-year breeders (two-year-olds) are most likely to produce really small eggs, 400g or less. By the following season, the eggs produced will in most cases be larger. An egg can be tiny and still hatch out a perfectly normal chick. It will of course also be very small, but will in many cases eventually catch up to the larger chicks.

2. **The Enormous Egg** - On the other end of the spectrum is the really huge egg, 700g or more, usually laid by a seasoned breeder. 550g is about the average egg weight among emus. There have been emu eggs laid that were over 1000g, but these are the exception rather than the rule and are sometimes due to the fusing of two eggs. Twins have occurred in such eggs, but survival rates were not good.

3. **The Torpedo- or Football-shaped Egg** - These eggs appear to have two pointed ends like a football, and it may be difficult to tell where the airspace is initially. It seems that this shape is also more difficult for the chick to maneuver in, since there is often a higher incidence of malpositioning in such eggs. In some cases elevating the airspace end of the egg slightly may help the chick get correctly oriented in the egg, reducing chances of malpositioning. Generally, the airspace of an egg is in the more rounded end, but since these eggs do not have a rounded end, the air space can be found after incubating the egg for a few days, by:

   (a) feeling with the cheek which end of the egg cools the fastest. This is the airspace end. OR:

   (b) placing egg on counter and observing which end tilts up more. This is the airspace end. It is easier to see towards end of incubation period.

Once the airspace end has been marked, a pad of gauze is placed under it to elevate it slightly and keep it elevated, even when trays tilt in the incubator during automatic turning. In an experiment done to determine whether emu eggs could be incubated in the vertical position, (turning through 45° each way) there were more malpositions recorded in this shape of egg. Even though the air space end was at the top, the chick's beak in most cases was at the other end and the body turned completely around. It is our opinion that this shape of emu egg should always be incubated in the horizontal position.

4. **The Ovoid Egg** - This type of egg has a distinctly pointed and distinctly rounded end, just like a chicken egg. They also tend to be shorter and fatter than football-shaped eggs. These eggs have been successfully incubated in the vertical position, turning at an angle of 45° each way, Some malpositions have been recorded, but not enough eggs have been incubated in this position yet to determine if the upright position was the reason for the chick malpositioning, or if this was due to some other factor(s). The economic advantage to being able to incubate some eggs upright would be that more eggs could be fitted into incubators. This in turn would mainly be a factor to consider if very expensive incubators were being used.

5. **The Lemon-shaped Egg** - Also a short fat egg, but with 2 pointed ends like a football-shaped egg. Again, it can be hard to tell which end is the airspace end at first.

6. **The Chalky or Aqua Egg** - Occasionally, an egg will be laid that is a beautiful light blue or aqua color and has a very dull or "chalky" finish. Generally, this type of egg passed out of the shell gland before receiving its final dark green coating and the shiny cuticle. (It may lose weight at a faster rate than normal.) Some aqua eggs have spent too long a time in the shell gland and have 1½ times as much shell as a normal egg. In cross-section, the egg-shell is white, aqua, dark green, then white, aqua again. These eggs often do not lose weight easily. Incubate under drier conditions if this is the case. Aqua eggs are worth incubating since they have been known to hatch normal, healthy chicks. Note, however, that due to the absence of a cuticle they are also more susceptible to bacterial infection and therefore to going rotten.

Chalky eggs that have spent longer than normal in the oviduct (e.g. 5 or 6 days) are often followed in the next 1 or 2 days by a soft-shelled egg. In these cases the soft-shelled egg is probably not due to any calcium deficiency but is simply the result of the "backup" caused by the chalky egg remaining in the oviduct for so long.

7. **The Soft-shelled or Thin-shelled Egg** - Encased only in membranes or in a very thin light green layer of shell, this type of egg usually did not spend enough time in the uterus (shell gland) to receive its full coatings of shell. It is often laid in conjunction with a chalky egg, as described above. Only if the condition persists is there cause for concern (see **Section 13.2**, "Problems in the Laying Hen").

8. **The Aqua-tipped Egg** - A normal looking, dark-green egg that has an aqua-colored area on one tip should also be marked "at-risk" for going rotten (like an aqua egg) since the final layer and cuticle are absent on the tip, allow-

ing easier access for bacteria. Incubate separately if possible (with other "at-risk" eggs), and monitor closely for any bad smell.

9. **The Cracked/Pecked Egg** - Any egg with a hole pecked in it all the way in to the egg contents is not worth incubating. The same goes for an egg that has frozen, whether it cracked as a result of this or not. Eggs with minor damage such as a very small crack/hole can be incubated after repairing the crack with glue/wax/nail varnish, but one should realize that bacteria may already have entered the egg and therefore it should be incubated as an "at-risk" egg for going rotten, in a separate incubator. Weight loss will also have to be monitored, as the egg may lose weight faster than it should.

10. **The Rotten Egg** - Fertility or infertility has nothing to do with whether an egg goes rotten or not. A rotten egg is simply one that has been invaded by bacteria. No chick can hatch out of a rotten egg, and in order not to cause problems to the other eggs (e.g. by oozing its contents through the pores out into the incubator, or worse, by exploding in the incubator) it should be removed as soon as it is detected. The immediate area should also be disinfected.

If an "eggy" smell is detected on first opening the incubator, instead of the normal, completely clean incubator smell, there is a rotten egg in the incubator. It can be detected by smelling each egg individually. Sometimes a rotten egg causes odor around it, so you may think you have found it when in fact you are smelling the egg next to it. To make sure, remove the suspected egg and then smell it again in a minute or two. It will, if anything, smell worse on cooling, and will also cool quickly since there is no developing chick in it to generate heat. If in doubt, separate the suspected egg from others but leave it in the incubator, and smell again the next day. It will soon be obvious which egg is rotten.

In the detection of rotten eggs, no instrument in the world is as effective as a good nose. A successful emu farmer makes as much use of the "sensors" with which God equipped him as he does the instruments provided by science and technology.

CHAPTER 10

Incubation and Hatching

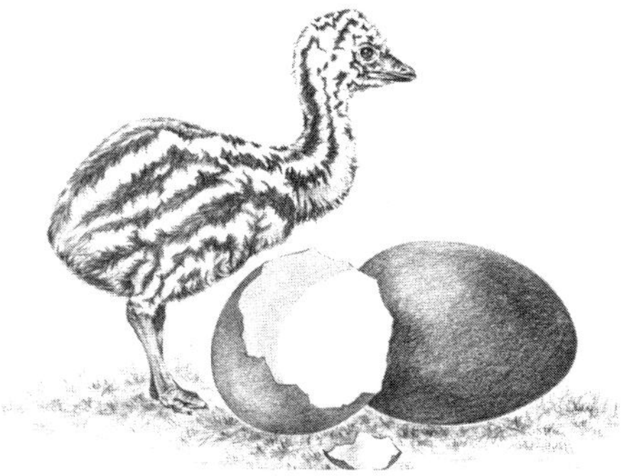

10.1 LIFE IN THE EGG

When a fertilized egg is incubated - whether artificially or naturally (by the parent), certain things begin to happen:

• Growth begins to take place in the small fertilized area at the top of the yolk, and it does not take long before the embryo becomes recognizable as a chick.

• A network of blood vessels begins to develop, spreading from embryo out over the yolk. The yolk sac is attached to the chick's gut via the navel. Out of the navel another membrane also grows, similar to the placenta of mammals. It is called the chorio-allantois, and it grows along the inside of the shell, eventually covering the entire inner shell membrane. Its plentiful supply of blood vessels enables it to carry oxygen to the embryo (diffused in via the shell pores) and to eliminate carbon dioxide, also by diffusion. It can also carry nutrients to the developing embryo via its blood supply, by the uptake of albumen as well as calcium from the shell itself. Finally, it stores the bird's excretory products. One or two small sacs of urates are generally a part of this very vascular membrane, which is seen to line the inner shell membrane after the chick has hatched (see **Plate 10.10** of color section.).

• The airspace enlarges, and the egg loses weight. (This is a mechanical process depending on several physical factors as outlined in **Section 10.5**, and is not dependent on whether or not there is life in the egg. Therefore an infertile egg will also show this characteristic.)

• Since the embryo is alive, it generates heat. As it grows, this becomes more and more noticeable until, a few days from hatching, it will feel hot to the touch and remain hot, where an infertile egg or dead-in-the-shell will rapidly cool on being removed from the incubator for a short while.

• Close to hatching, the embryo's oxygen needs increase greatly. He begins to move around in the shell a lot, and begins to draw the yolk sac up into his body. The inner shell membrane begins to lie down over his body as his struggling separates it from the outer shell membrane.This stage is known as "drawdown", and can sometimes be detected by tapping (see **Section 10.4**). Soon after this the chick breaks through the inner membrane into the air space (internal pip). He may rest a while, then within 1 to 3 days he pips the shell.

Fig. 10.1 - Stages in the development of the chick inside the egg.

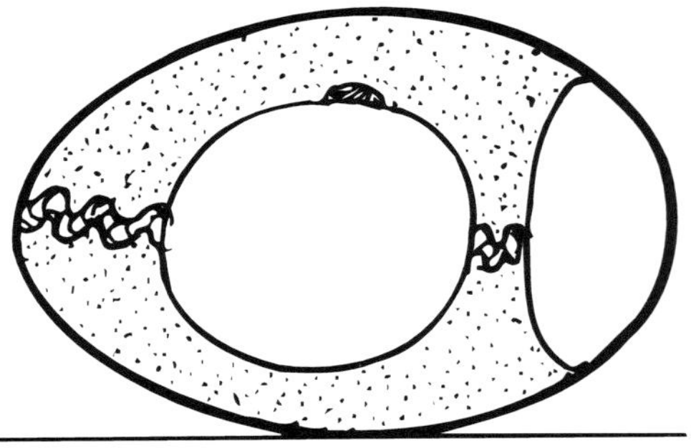

A. Freshly laid egg with fertilized blastodisc (on top of yolk). Egg not tilted.

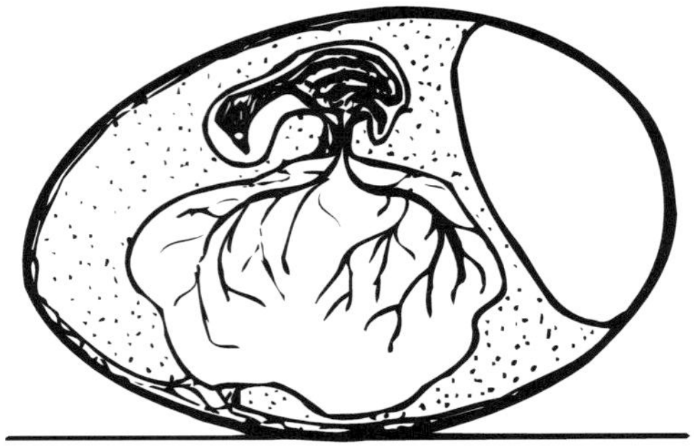

B. Embryo growing. Blood vessels growing over yolk sac. Chorio-allantois growing from chick's navel down onto sides of egg. Enlarging air space causing slight tilt to egg.

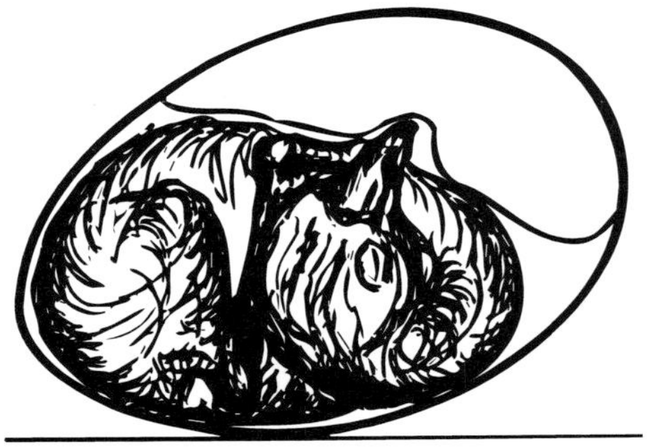

C. Chick just prior to internal pip. Inner membrane starting to lie down over chick. Air space causing very noticeable tilt to egg.

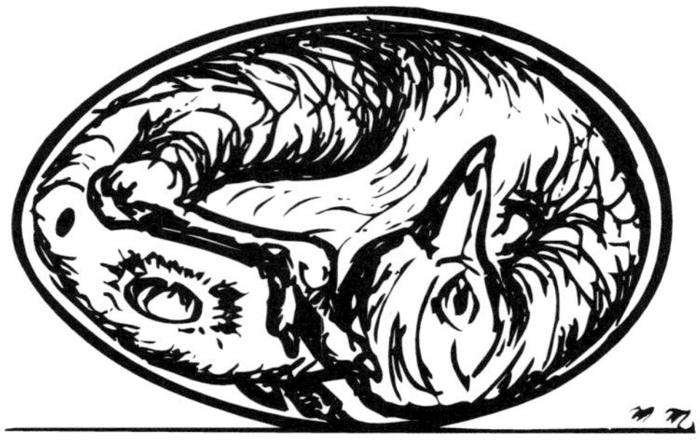

D. Chick in hatching position, having pipped internally and now occupying the entire space of the egg. Yolk sac almost all drawn in through navel. Egg no longer tilted.

Some chicks will hatch out completely within a few hours after pipping, others take as long as 2 days. Either is normal, and no human intervention is necessary unless the chick becomes disoriented and slips his beak and head away from the opening and back down into the egg. On the rare occasions that this happens it may become necessary to remove a few extra pieces of shell so the chick does not suffocate.

10.2 THE INCUBATOR

An incubator is a machine used to artificially hatch eggs by the application of heat to them. There are 2 types of incubators: Still-air, which only have one tray and which simulate the conditions under the laying hen (i.e. the warmest air rises to the top and eggs are cooler underneath) and forced-air incubators in which a fan blows to distribute heat evenly over all the eggs. Forced-air incubators can have several trays stacked above one another, and are the kind used in all commercial hatching operations. Still-air incubators are used for small batches of eggs, e.g. in schools and for demonstration purposes.

Because in still-air incubators there is quite a large temperature variation between the top and the bottom, these incubators are generally set at a higher temperature than forced-air incubators. This is where confusion as to temperature settings will sometimes arise. Provided the manufacturer of the incubator has done his homework on the particular species of bird eggs to be incubated, the manufacturer's instructions should be followed.

Turning of eggs is necessary no matter what type of incubator is used. Birds turn their eggs frequently by shuffling them from side to side. Most commercial incubators have automatic turning devices which turn the egg trays as frequently as every hour, although eggs will also hatch successfully if turned as little as 2 to 3 times a day

Trays of water placed on the top shelf of the incubator are generally used if the humidity needs to be raised. Some incubators have more sophisticated built-in humidity control systems. These generally also have built-in sensors to measure the humidity and give a percentage readout. Humidity levels can also be raised by closing the vent holes, usually located at the back of the incubator, but this is not recommended in the incubation of emu eggs as the danger of insufficient air circulation then becomes too high. Most emu eggs are incubated with vent holes completely open. Besides, lower humidity levels are usually called for in emu egg incubation compared with poultry or other commercially hatched birds, so open vents are more appropriate for this reason also.

10.3 THE INCUBATION PROCESS

Equipment

To successfully incubate and hatch emu eggs, the following equipment will be needed:

- Good incubator, with accurate thermometer and preferably equipped with automatic turner.
- Hatcher, with accurate thermometer
- Formaldehyde, to clean incubator and hatcher prior to incubation.
- Standby generator (or access to one) in case of power failure
- Short metal rod for egg-tapping, to determine when an egg should be moved to the hatcher. (In other species of birds whose eggs are not opaque like the emu, **candling** is an alternative.)

- Accurate scale measuring in single-gram increments (at least) if egg weight loss is going to be monitored. Note that an inaccurate scale is worse than no scale at all, since it may lead to making the wrong humidity adjustment.

- Hygrometer wick for taking wet-bulb readings (unless incubator is already fitted with the appropriate instruments for measuring humidity).

- Brooder boxes for keeping new chicks in as well as some clip-on lamps to keep them warm.

- Betadine solution and ointment for navels.

- Disinfectant solution which is safe for use around eggs and chicks - use for cleaning in and around hatcher/incubator as needed, misting in air, etc.

- Well-laid-out chart or book or computer program for record-keeping (see **Table 10.1**). In addition to these detailed egg charts showing the egg/chick production of individual pairs of birds, most emu farmers also keep a daily journal in which the number and date of each egg is recorded as it is laid, along with the number/name of the parent birds, due date, and hatch date.

Best results are achieved when the incubator is placed in a climate-controlled environment, i.e. an air conditioned/heated (as needed) room which maintains a temperature of about 70°F to 78°F. An incubator cannot lower temperature if the room gets too hot; it is only designed to produce heat. Central air conditioning is of course ideal, but window units in the incubator room work fine too, provided they provide adequate ventilation. In the latter case, fans and venting to the outside may be needed to improve actual air circulation.

A good thermometer can have two functions: for taking dry-bulb readings and for wet-bulb readings. The dry-bulb reading is simply the normal temperature reading at which the incubator is set. The wet-bulb reading, or "hygrometer reading", is achieved by placing one end of a hygrometer wick into a small bottle of water and, once wet through, threading the other end over the thermometer. The thermometer's bulb or probe is of course inside the incubator while the temperature is read from the outside, after closing the incubator door. After about10 minutes, the temperature will have dropped to a certain point and will remain there. This is the wet-bulb reading. By comparing dry-bulb and wet-bulb temperatures on a special chart (see **Table 10.5**), percentage relative humidity can also be found. The drop in temperature of the wet-bulb reading is caused by cooling by evaporation, which continues until an equilibrium is reached. The drier the air, the greater the rate of evaporation and the lower the reading will be. For as long as the wick remains wet and provided there are no changes in humidity such as adding a pan of water, the wet-bulb reading will remain constant at that point. Use distilled water to prolong the life of the wick. Other absorbent material such as a piece of lace from a running shoe can be used in place of a hygrometer wick, if need be.

Table 10.1 - Example of egg record-keeping chart for use in incubation.

EGG #					
DATE LAID					
DATE INCUB.					
WEATHER CONDITIONS					
EGG CONDITION					
EGG TREATMENTS					
INCUBATOR CONDITIONS					
INITIAL WEIGHT /DATE					
WT./DATE					
WT./DATE					
WT./DATE					
DATE DUE (50d.)					
DATE SOUNDED					
DATE HATCHED					
RESULTS					

Preparing the incubator and hatcher

Before the eggs are placed in it, the incubator should be:

- Scrubbed clean, using water with disinfectant (e.g. chlorine bleach).
- Fumigated with formaldehyde (obtainable from local pharmacy). Mix 1 part formaldehyde, 10 parts water and spray this mixture all over inside of incubator, trays and separators. Do not inhale fumes as formaldehyde is very poisonous. Keep children and animals away, turn incubator(s) and hatcher on, open windows of room for ventilation and allow 12-24 hours for the poisonous gases to dissipate. This will kill any micro-organisms present in incubators and hatcher.

Note: it is advisable to fumigate even a brand-new incubator, since just because it looks clean does not mean there are no micro-organisms lurking in it. Fumigation should be done prior to every breeding season, and more often if there seems to be a problem with contamination by bacteria/fungi etc. Eggs should be removed prior to fumigation. In some poultry hatcheries it is common practice to fumigate actual eggs, but the effects of fumigating emu eggs with formaldehyde have not yet been studied enough to make this a recommended practice. Under most reasonably sanitary conditions of egg handling and incubation, a good hatch can be achieved without egg fumigation. Possibly it could prove of benefit once operations reach the much larger commercial level. Formalin and potassium permanganate crystals may also be used for fumigation, as they will release formaldehyde gas when combined.

- Turned on for a few days and periodically checked to ensure it is holding the correct temperature. Any adjustments to the thermostat should be made before eggs are introduced, so that it is running at a constant temperature by the time eggs are placed in it. (Follow manufacturer's instructions for setting thermostats.) An accurate extra thermometer with a probe and a long cord is extremely useful for placement in different parts of the incubator, in order to ensure that there is not a great deal of temperature variation between top and bottom, or back and front of the incubator. Temperature should not vary by more than ½°F either side of the set temperature. A good incubator will distribute heat evenly. Uneven heat distribution can also mean that the air flow is uneven, i.e. some parts of the incubator are not as well ventilated as others. This could cause poor development or even death in the eggs situated in those parts of the incubator.

- Checked to make sure the automatic turner is working.

The hatcher is treated in exactly the same way, except that there will be no automatic turner to check. If an incubator is to be used as a hatcher, level the trays, pull them forward a little to rest on the front bars for support, and make sure the automatic turner is off (so as not to strain and break the mechanism). If the incubator is not equipped with separators for eggs, these can be made very easily by bending chicken-wire into a "W" shape lengthways and fitting a piece into each tray. In this way, eggs can be arranged in rows along the length of the tray and will be held steady when the trays turn, rather than rolling around and bumping into one another. Another advantage is that chicken-wire can be easily bent to accommodate a very large or very small egg, unlike "standard" wire separators which have similar-sized compartments. The use of wire rather than solid materials to separate eggs permits airflow to remain uninterrupted, which is important. The separators are of course fumigated with the rest of the machine.

Loading (setting) the eggs

Eggs are usually marked and weighed prior to being incubated. After the appropriate information has been recorded, the incubator trays are levelled and the

Table 10.2 - Quick-reference hatch date table. (50 days)

DATE INCUBATED	DATE DUE	DATE INCUBATED	DATE DUE	DATE INCUBATED	DATE DUE	DATE INCUBATED	DATE DUE
OCT. 1	NOV. 20	DEC. 1	JAN. 20	FEB. 1	MAR. 23	APR. 1	MAY21
2	21	2	21	2	24	2	22
3	22	3	22	3	25	3	23
4	23	4	23	4	26	4	24
5	24	5	24	5	27	5	25
6	25	6	25	6	28	6	26
7	26	7	26	7	29	7	27
8	27	8	27	8	30	8	28
9	28	9	28	9	31	9	29
10	29	10	29	10	APR. 1	10	30
11	30	11	30	11	2	11	31
12	DEC. 1	12	31	12	3	12	JUN. 1
13	2	13	FEB. 1	13	4	13	2
14	3	14	2	14	5	14	3
15	4	15	3	15	6	15	4
16	5	16	4	16	7	16	5
17	6	17	5	17	8	17	6
18	7	18	6	18	9	18	7
19	8	19	7	19	10	19	8
20	9	20	8	20	11	20	9
21	10	21	9	21	12	21	10
22	11	22	10	22	13	22	11
23	12	23	11	23	14	23	12
24	13	24	12	24	15	24	13
25	14	25	13	25	16	25	14
26	15	26	14	26	17	26	15
27	16	27	15	27	18	27	16
28	17	28	16	*28	19	28	17
29	18	29	17			29	18
30	19	30	18			30	19
31	20	31	19				

DATE INCUBATED	DATE DUE	DATE INCUBATED	DATE DUE	DATE INCUBATED	DATE DUE	DATE INCUBATED	DATE DUE
NOV. 1	DEC. 21	JAN. 1	FEB. 20	MAR. 1	APR. 20	MAY. 1	JUN.20
2	22	2	21	2	21	2	21
3	23	3	22	3	22	3	22
4	24	4	23	4	23	4	23
5	25	5	24	5	24	5	24
6	26	6	25	6	25	6	25
7	27	7	26	7	26	7	26
8	28	8	27	8	27	8	27
9	29	9	28	9	28	9	28
10	30	*10	MAR. 1	10	29	10	29
11	31	11	2	11	30	11	30
12	JAN. 1	12	3	12	MAY 1	12	JUL. 1
13	2	13	4	13	2	13	2
14	3	14	5	14	3	14	3
15	4	15	6	15	4	15	4
16	5	16	7	16	5	16	5
17	6	17	8	17	6	17	6
18	7	18	9	18	7	18	7
19	8	19	10	19	8	19	8
20	9	20	11	20	9	20	9
21	10	21	12	21	10	21	10
22	11	22	13	22	11	22	11
23	12	23	14	23	12	23	12
24	13	24	15	24	13	24	13
25	14	25	16	25	14	25	14
26	15	26	17	26	15	26	15
27	16	27	18	27	16	27	16
28	17	28	19	28	17	28	17
29	18	29	20	29	18	29	18
30	19	30	21	30	19	30	19
		31	22	31	20	31	20

* Note that in a leap year, any eggs incubated between January 10 and February 29 will show a difference by ONE DAY (less) in the due date. From March 1, the table is the same for any year.

eggs are placed in them in such a way as to evenly balance the tray (this puts less strain on the turning mechanism.) Emu eggs are usually placed horizontally rather than vertically, and they should be positioned to rotate from side to side, not end to end.

There has been some experimentation with setting eggs in the vertical position. This does not of course mean that they actually spend the incubation period standing on end, since the trays always rest in such a position that the egg is in approximately the same position as if it were lying on its side. However, it does mean that the rotation takes place through the vertical rather than through the horizontal axis of the egg. In poultry eggs, the sole reason for incubating eggs in this position is to fit more eggs in the incubator, which makes economic sense considering the large numbers involved in commercial poultry operations. Controversy exists as to whether this position causes fewer malpositioned chicks or not, since the positioning of the egg is not the only contributing factor to chick malpositioning. In the limited data available on emu eggs incubated in this position, there was some success, but in "football-shaped" eggs this position appeared to cause a higher incidence of malpositioning, with chicks that were turned completely backwards in the egg.

Any egg that is to be incubated in the vertical position should be placed with the air space end up. Since it is not possible with some emu eggs to know which end is the air space end until after a day or so of incubation (see **Section 9.3**), provision still has to be made for some incubation in the horizontal position as well.

Those who argue that the horizontal position would cause more malpositions

Table 10.3 - Emu incubation periods at different temperatures.

Temperature	Average number of days to hatch	
96.0°F(35.5°C)	55 - 56 days	
96.5°F (35.8°C)	52 - 54 days	OPTIMUM HATCH RESULTS
97.0°F (36.1°C)	50 - 52 days	OPTIMUM HATCH RESULTS
97.5°F (36.4°C)	49 - 51 days	OPTIMUM HATCH RESULTS
98.0°F (36.7°C)	46 - 48 days	

than the vertical position should remember that in Nature, emu eggs are always incubated in the horizontal position. The shape of the egg does not lend itself to remaining in any other position, unlike rounded or more ovoid eggs of other species of birds. Therefore, it is not likely that you will go very far wrong by choosing the same incubation position as the one seen in Nature. The good results obtained by many emu farmers in different areas testify to this.

Temperature and humidity settings

The most commonly used temperature for the incubation of emu eggs is 97.5°F. As can be seen from **Table 10.3**, this is not the ONLY temperature at which emu eggs can be successfully incubated. Incubation temperature, like so many other factors affecting life, does have certain parameters or limits within which healthy development is still possible. Towards the upper and lower limits, however, more problems are likely to be seen.

The temperature of 97.5°F has been used successfully at altitudes from sea level to 7000'. However, from the limited data available on the incubation of emu eggs at high altitudes, it appears that humidity levels there may have to be slightly higher - although as always, egg weight loss should be the chief determining factor in setting humidity. Airflow must be excellent since air contains less oxygen at higher altitudes.

To start with, a humidity setting of 70°F - 75°F (24% to 35%) at the above temperature can be used. These settings provide for adequate weight loss in most emu eggs. Due to differences in egg porosity, some eggs will lose weight at faster or slower rates than others under the same conditions, and if these come dangerously close to the upper or lower limit of the "safe range" (see **Section 10.5** on Weight Loss in Emu Eggs), they may need to be incubated in a different incubator with the appropriate humidity setting. If there is no extra incubator, any eggs that need a higher humidity may be incubated in the hatcher and turned by hand. Turning should be done 3 times daily and should be done back and forth, not the same direction each time.

The hatcher, into which the eggs are moved when they have "sounded" (usually 1 to 4 days before the end of the incubation period) is usually set either at the same temperature as the incubator or one degree lower. The chick at this point is filling up almost the entire egg and making strenuous efforts to muscle his way out of it.

Table 10.4 - Incubation Temperature Conversions

°F	°C
96.0	35.55
96.5	35.8
97.0	36.1
97.5	36.4
98.0	36.66
98.5	36.9

Formulae for Temperature Conversions:

$°C = (°F - 32) \times 5/9$

$°F = (°C \times 9/5) + 32$

Once in the hatcher, the egg need no longer be turned as this might disorient the chick which is trying to hatch. Usually, the chick will first make a hole in the shell with his beak (external pip). After a short rest period he appears to push with the back of his neck while bracing with one foot in or near the hole made by the beak. Eventually he cracks the shell either longitudinally or as in most cases, by pushing the top part right off (from the crack made by pipping) and crawls out. He will usually be slightly damp but usually dries off within the hour. There is no significant weight loss in the chick between hatch and drying out; the first significant weight loss comes after the first (dark green) stool has been passed, and can be between 8 and 24g as recorded to date.

Unless a problem is seen or suspected, there is no reason to "help" a chick out of the shell once he has pipped. After all, he now has everything he needs - food from the yolk sac, and plenty of air - so he is in no danger. Any extra time in the egg is helpful in ensuring that the navel will be completely closed on hatch, lessening the danger of bacterial contamination through an incompletely closed navel. It is still a good precaution to put Betadine on the navel, however.

The humidity level in the hatcher is probably not as critical as the humidity during incubation. This is very likely the reason why some farmers have good hatch results with no water pans at all in the hatcher, using the same wet-bulb reading as in the incubator (70-74°F) whereas others place a large pan of water in the hatcher to achieve a wet-bulb reading of around 84°F and also have a successful hatch. Poultry hatcheries raise the humidity in hatchers in order to prevent chicks from sticking to drying shell membranes. This does not seem to be much of a problem in emus, since the white inner membrane which lies on the chick generally becomes brittle and thin on drying, and tends to fall off readily. The membrane will usually dry in this way even in the more humid conditions (84°F). It is probably safe to say that emu chicks can pip and hatch under rather a large range of humidity levels. Time spent in the hatcher is very minimal compared to the long period spent in the incubator. Thus if the incubation conditions were optimal, chances are there will be no problems with hatching. By the same token, optimum temperature and humidity conditions in the hatcher will

Table 10.5 - Percentage relative humidity at various wet-bulb/dry-bulb temperatures.

Wet-Bulb Temperature (°F)	Dry -Bulb Temperature (°F) 96°	97°	98°
67°	21%	19%	18%
68°	23%	21%	20%
69°	25%	23%	22%
70°	27%	25%	24%
71°	29%	27%	26%
72°	31%	29%	28%
73°	33%	32%	30%
74°	35%	34%	32%
75°	38%	36%	34%
76°	40%	38%	36%
77°	42%	41%	39%
78°	45%	43%	41%
79°	47%	45%	43%
80°	50%	48%	46%
81°	53%	50%	48%
82°	55%	53%	51%
83°	58%	56%	53%
84°	61%	58%	56%
85°	64%	61%	59%
86°	67%	64%	62%
87°	70%	67%	64%

not make up for improper conditions of incubation. Unless oxygen levels in the hatcher are too low, any chick deaths at or just before pipping are probably due to problems in incubating, not problems in the hatcher. Many a farmer blames himself for a pre-hatch death, thinking he could have saved the chick had he opened the shell and assisted the chick. In many cases this is not true; the egg may simply not have lost enough weight or had enough oxygen during incubation.

Water pans to be used in the hatcher should have a few drops of disinfectant added to prevent growth of bacteria/fungi.

Because the humidity of the air is so high in many parts of the U.S., in particular the central and southern areas, it is often not necessary to add any water pans to incubators in order to maintain correct humidity levels, even in air-conditioned houses or rooms. (Water is often added to hatchers, however.) In drier areas or at higher altitudes, water pans are usually needed both in incubators and hatchers to attain the desired levels. To increase humidity, increase surface area of water trays (not depth).

Monitoring Eggs Due to Hatch

The vigor and movement seen in hatching eggs (both before and after pip) will often greatly increase when the egg is cooled (by taking it out of the incubator for weighing, or just by opening incubator door), as well as when the egg is spoken/whistled to, or tapped. All these factors seem to act as stimuli for the chick to increase his hatching efforts. Of course, eggs should not be held out of the hatcher for too long, but some stimulation every few hours does seem to encourage the chick to hatch. By pressing the egg to the ear and whistling to it, an answering cheep is frequently heard once the chick is through into the airspace. He is now breathing via his lungs rather than via diffusion through shell to the blood vessels of the chorioallantois. Very occasionally a chick may be heard to cheep before he has pipped internally, but generally, hearing chirping is a good indication that the chick has in fact broken through. "Sounding" along with the level position of the egg (see **Fig. 10.1(d)**) will confirm this. The chick's movements can also be felt. Some farmers use a stethoscope to listen to eggs, but the ear alone will suffice.

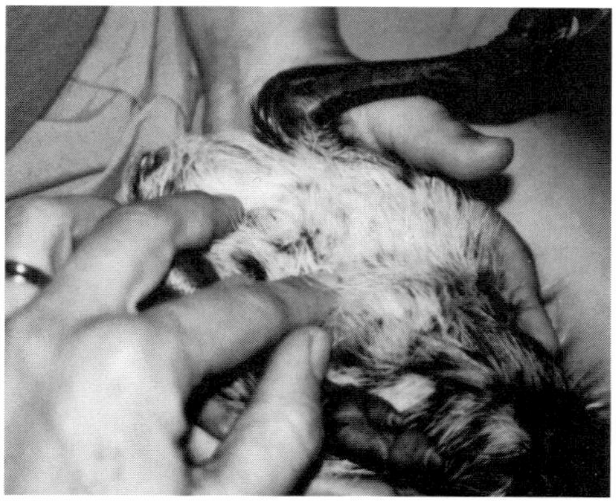

Plate 10.1 - Newly hatched chick with navel nicely closed.

It is interesting to note that the position in which the egg is placed in the incubator (as indicated by the number visible on the top part of the egg) is usually also the position in which it hatches. If the egg is placed on a flat surface several days prior to hatching and rolled one way or the other, it will always settle back into one position as dictated by its center of gravity, and this is usually with its number on the top surface as during incubation. **Fig. 10.1(c)** shows the position of the growing chick in relation to the air space during this time.

In case of power failure, a standby generator is invaluable. Power failure not only causes eggs to lose heat, but may also cause a buildup of carbon dioxide to dangerous levels in the incubator, since the air is no longer being vented. For this reason, vents should still be left wide open during a power failure. Loss of power for more than an hour will probably have a detrimental effect on the hatchability of the eggs, depending on their stage of incubation.

Eggs should never be transported after the incubation process has started, as this can cause many losses.

10.4 EGG TAPPING

Since emu eggs are completely opaque and therefore cannot be candled like most other eggs, a different method must be used to determine when an egg should be moved from the incubator to the hatcher. (Candling involves shining a strong light through an egg after it has been incubating for a while, to check if the egg is fertile, to monitor changes in the size of the airspace, and to check when internal pip has taken place.) Egg-tapping is a simple, quick and convenient way of determining when "internal pip" has taken place, and therefore when the egg should be moved to the hatcher.

An "egg tapper" can be any piece of fairly heavy metal, such as steel or iron, that is in the form of a short rod about 6 or 7 inches long. Hold it loosely in an "overhand" grip as illustrated (**Fig. 10.2**) and pull out the tray of eggs to be tapped, after first levelling the trays in the incubator, of course. Give each egg two or three quick, short taps in the middle of the egg, tapping with your wrist as loose and flexible as if you were playing a drum, and with about the same vigor. Too soft a tap will not give a good "sounding". The reason for doing several eggs in quick succession is for the purpose of comparing sounds; the "hollow" sound of an egg where the chick has broken through the inner membrane (internal pip) will be a very different one from all the eggs where this has not yet taken place.

The test to determine whether you are tapping correctly, if you have never had this method demonstrated to you, is to place a hollow, blown-out (infertile) emu egg in the tray next to the others. Make sure this "test egg" is disinfected first, of course. It should be dry, clean, and have a hole in one end only. Tap on some of the eggs that you know are not anywhere close to hatching; then tap on the hollow egg. There should be a distinct difference in sound. Interestingly enough, for some reason to do with the acoustics in the egg, this hollow egg will sound almost exactly the same as an egg in which internal pip has taken place.

With practice, it also becomes possible to hear by tapping when "drawdown" in the egg is starting to take place. Up to this point, the inner membrane has been concavely stretched like a diaphragm between the growing chick and the air space. Prior to internal pip, the vigorous movements of the chick will usually cause the inner membrane to detach somewhat from the egg walls and lie down over the chick, following its contours. When this "drawdown" occurs, the acoustics in the egg will be changed somewhat.

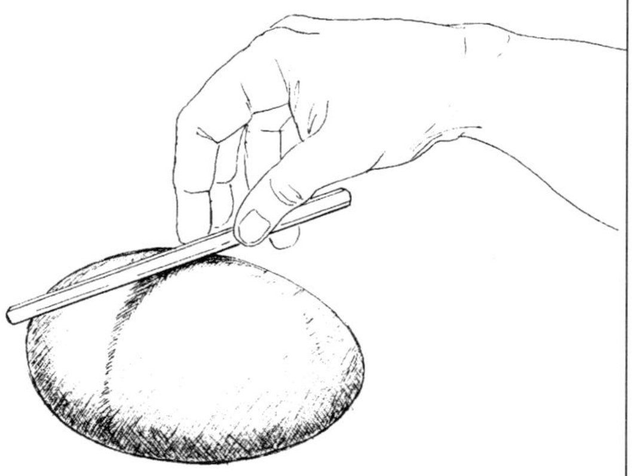

Fig. 10.2 - Tapping the egg.

The most drastic change in sound, however, occurs at internal pip when the chick's beak has broken through the membrane and into the egg's airspace.

The reason why egg-tapping is so useful to the emu farmer is that he will in all probability be incubating eggs of many different sizes and shapes, from different pairs of birds. Because of these differences, there may be variations in time periods to hatch by as much as two or three days, even though the eggs are incubated under the same conditions. Some may be a little earlier than expected, some a little later. By tapping every day from about the 40th day of incubation, any sound changes can be detected early and the possibility of a chick hatching in the incubator and falling out of a tray can be avoided.

In the commercial incubation of poultry eggs, turkey eggs or any other type of bird that has been domesticated for a longer period of time, selective breeding has produced birds of greater uniformity within each breed. This also leads to a more uniform type of egg. In addition, any eggs that deviate from the normal (e.g. smaller, larger, misshapen, rough-textured) are usually discarded prior to incubation. In this way, commercial hatcheries can be sure most of the chicks will hatch on the same day. Emu farming is not yet at the stage where eggs that differ from the "average" are discarded; rather, all eggs are incubated. Therefore greater differences in incubation periods are to be expected although more uniformity is certainly something to strive for in the future.

When the egg has "sounded"

Once an egg has "sounded" properly (that is, it sounds distinctly hollow on tapping) this usually means that it will be able to hatch with no problems, provided it is placed in a hatcher with excellent air flow and the proper temperature. By the time an egg "sounds", there will also be other signs that it contains a vigorous, healthy chick: the egg will jiggle if placed on a flat surface, especially if talked to or whistled to; scrabbling movements will be felt inside the egg, and pecking may be heard if placed next to the ear; the egg will feel quite hot to the touch, especially if pressed to the cheek or other temperature-sensitive area of one's body; and chirping may be heard, especially in response to talking or whistling. Since the chick now fills up most of the egg, an air space (cool area) can no longer be felt when holding the egg to the cheek. The egg will feel hot almost all over.

The period between "sounding" and hatch is variable. It may be as little as a few hours or as much as 2 or 3 days. It is better not to get impatient but rather allow the chick to pip on its own; but if there is a previous history of suffocation in the shell just prior to hatching in eggs laid by the same hen, it is safe to make a small hole in what was the airspace side once an egg has sounded. The beak should be visible, having broken through the membrane. There is now no further cause for alarm: the chick has everything it needs, i.e. warmth, food (from its yolk sac) and oxygen, and it will get out of the egg by itself in its own time. Nothing can be gained by hurrying it, in most cases. There are just a few hatching situations that do need some assistance, and these are covered in **Section 10.7**.

The "porcelain-sounding" egg

Although it is not usually possible to tell by tapping whether an egg is fertile or not (until it is close to hatching and "sounds", of course) there are some infertile eggs that will produce a different sound altogether on tapping. It is a "tinny" sound very much like tapping on porcelain or china, and is generally heard when the egg is infertile but the membrane separating the airspace from the egg contents is no longer stretched, but has become flaccid. Sometimes this occurs because the egg is busy going rotten. However, some thoroughly rotten eggs never sound "tinny" - although they can of course always be detected by smell. In any case, a tinny-sounding egg has never in our experience produced a live chick. If one is not sure about the sound, it may be wise to place this egg in a separate "problem egg" incubator until its due date. After the due date, it can be opened to confirm the original diagnosis. With practice, one will become more sure about the status of these eggs and can open and discard such eggs earlier, to make more room in the incubator for viable eggs.

10.5 WEIGHT LOSS IN EMU EGGS

Introduction

All bird eggs lose weight during incubation. They cannot gain weight, because the egg is a sealed package into which nothing except air can enter. The growth of the embryo into a chick is merely a transfer process, as egg yolk and albumen are used up to make the chick's muscles, organs and bones. A small amount of carbon dioxide and water vapor are lost in the normal process of respiration, but the main reason for weight loss in eggs is that the egg is porous in order to be able to take up oxygen from the air, and this also enables evaporation of moisture from the egg to take place. Since this is a purely mechanical factor that depends on the egg's environment, and is not something that the developing embryo can control, one can understand how important correct humidity settings are. In order to control weight loss in emu eggs, therefore, one simply needs to control the rate of evaporation.

There are several factors that have an influence on the rate of evaporation. They include: **temperature** (the higher the temperature, the faster the rate of evaporation); **humidity** (the lower the humidity of the surrounding air, the faster the rate of evaporation) and **air flow** (the greater the air flow, the faster the rate of evaporation.) Anyone who has ever hung out sheets to dry on a line will know that the quickest drying period (i.e. evaporation of moisture from the sheets) is experienced under hot, dry, windy conditions. An additional factor which may have a small influence on evaporation due to its effect on air pressure, is **altitude**.

Other than these general factors influencing evaporation, eggs have some specific factors which will cause some eggs to evaporate moisture at different rates to others. The main factor is **egg porosity**, which is influenced by shell thickness and sizes/numbers of pores. However, the size and shape of an egg may also have some effect, as discussed below.

Egg size, shape, texture and color: Possible effects on weight loss

- **Size** - Larger eggs often tend to lose weight slightly less rapidly than smaller ones.

- **Shape** - A sphere has the smallest possible evaporating surface in relation to its volume. The less spherical the egg, the greater its evaporating surface (e.g. long, football-shaped eggs will usually lose weight at a faster rate than rounder or more ovoid ones, which have the same volume but a relatively smaller evaporating surface).

- **Texture** - If one were to categorize textures as grapefruit, orange, lemon and lime, with lime being the smoothest and grapefruit the most pitted, usually smoother eggs will lose weight faster. "Gritty" textures, however, will also usually lose weight faster and this type of texture indicates incomplete or disturbed shell formation - hen may have a dietary deficiency or inflamed oviduct.

- **Color** - the more light green flecks scattered throughout the egg, generally the higher the rate of weight loss. A very dark green egg usually loses weight at a slower rate. Eggs that are unevenly colored e.g. very speckled (light green) at air space end may have variable rates of weight loss, since the uneven texture can indicate incomplete or disturbed shell formation, like the gritty texture. The two often go together.

INTERRELATIONSHIP: All of these factors are interrelated and one factor cannot be considered without taking the others into account, since they all make up the egg. They should serve as guidelines only. The best method for proper incubation management is egg weighing.

Egg Weight Loss: General Information

- If humidity is fairly constant, weight loss usually is at a constant rate. Therefore, if an egg loses 1.5 grams in one day, it should lose about the same the next day, and so forth. After 4 days, this egg should have lost 4 x 1.5g = 6 grams.
- Total weight loss is usually expressed as a percentage of the egg's original weight. (This is of course because every egg has a different weight.)
- Normal parameters (limits) within which emu eggs can be successfully hatched vary between 10 - 20%. The ideal would be in the middle, i.e. 13 - 17 %. Deaths may occur at either extreme, i.e. 10% and less, or 20% and more. Obviously, there will always be some exceptions that do survive these extremes.
- Each hen usually lays similar eggs which follow a similar weight loss pattern. Therefore, if you lost the first two eggs from a hen because of too high weight loss (say 24 %), you can usually assume that her other eggs will follow the same pattern, and incubate them all at a higher humidity. (Double-check by weighing). Exception to this rule might be the hen who lays gritty or inconsistently colored/textured eggs. These may also show inconsistent weight loss, e.g. one egg normal, the next too high.

Using Egg Weighing To Help Prevent Problems Before They Occur

If you weigh an egg only at the beginning and at the end of incubation, find a dead, dehydrated chick and calculate that the egg lost 21% of its original weight (too high), it may already be too late for many of the hen's other eggs that are soon due to hatch. If, on the other hand, you weigh eggs daily for the first 3 or 4 days, calculate how much weight the egg should be losing and compare this with how much it is losing, you can take preventive measures if there seems to be a problem, and be able to successfully hatch many chicks that would otherwise have died.

Example: Your egg weighs 500 g. Calculate the ideal weight loss as 15%.

15% x 500g = 75 grams (total "target" weight loss.)

If you are incubating at 97.5°F, you can estimate that the egg should hatch in about 50 days.

$$\text{Target DAILY weight loss} = \frac{75 \text{ grams}}{50} = 1.5 \text{ grams/day}$$

To calculate the "danger zone", find the target daily weight loss at 10% and at 20% by the same method.

10% loss gives a 1 g daily weight loss. (too low)

20% loss gives a 2 g daily weight loss. (too high)

Therefore, if after 4 days the egg has already lost 10 grams, this means the daily weight loss was 2.5 g , which is even more than the 20% weight loss line. The egg can be saved by one or more of the following methods:

1. Increase humidity, e.g. by incubating in a separate incubator with large tray of water, or in the more humid hatcher if no spare incubator is available. (Eggs incubated in hatcher will have to be hand turned three times daily).

2. Lower temperature slightly. This also helps reduce the rate of evaporation, although it may cause the egg to hatch a little later by a day or so.

3. If egg is still losing moisture at too high a rate, paint the egg in longitudinal or crosswise stripes. (Do not cover whole egg with paint, and use non-toxic paint e.g. acrylic textile paint.) This will seal some of the pores (slowing evaporation) but not all (so egg can still get oxygen). Air flow must be excellent for this method to work well. Chicks do not seem to have any problems hatching out of painted eggs.

At the other end of the scale, if eggs are losing too little weight, methods that may help include dehumidifying the air, raising temperature slightly to increase evaporation, but perhaps most importantly, increasing air flow and fresh air exchange.

NB: To help save time and labor in percentage weight loss calculations, the Egg Weight Loss Chart has been provided (**Table 10.6**). Its use is outlined further on in the text.

Erratic Weight Loss

Great fluctuations in humidity are almost as bad for a developing embryo as great fluctuations in temperature. An uninsulated incubator which has no automatic humidity control and is not in a climate-controlled environment will have fluctuations in humidity according to the (weather) conditions around it. This means the embryo is constantly having to adjust to different rates of evaporation, and its body metabolism may not be able to cope. Embryonic death or a weak, problem chick could result. For good hatchability, egg weight loss must be kept fairly constant, by keeping humidity constant. A **total** weight loss of 15% in an egg does not necessarily mean the weight loss **rate** (daily loss) was correct: if the egg lost the last 10% in the last 10 days of incubation, the weight loss rate for the first 40 days was obviously not sufficient. Damage has already been done, and increasing the rate of evaporation the last few days in an attempt to reach "target" will not undo this damage.

Using the Egg Weight Loss Chart (Table 10.6)

The Egg Weight Loss Chart (**Table 10.6**) is intended as a guide only, bearing in mind that an egg is a living thing and will have certain parameters (limits) within which it can successfully hatch. It is also important to remember that all factors affecting incubation are interrelated. Thus, it does no good to have correct weight loss rate in eggs if the temperature is completely wrong, or there is not enough air flow, or the eggs are not being turned, or are jarred greatly on turning. Pre-incubation problems, such as wet/muddy eggs which may have become infected, or eggs that have been held in storage for too long or stored under the wrong conditions, will also have an effect on egg hatchability, no matter how correctly the eggs are incubated.

In the Egg Weight Loss Chart, all figures are in grams. "Final Weight" is expressed to the nearest gram. "Daily Loss" is expressed to 2 decimal places. All weight loss figures have been calculated on the basis of 50 days incubation. Variations by a couple of days on either side of this will not make a significant difference, and the figures can still be used as a guideline in these cases.

For the sake of clarity and convenience, only 3 different percentage weight losses have been recorded: 13%, 15% and 17%. This provides a quick reference as well as a good basis for estimates of any percentages in between.

To use the chart, follow this procedure:

1. Weigh the egg just before placing in incubator, using a good, accurate scale which measures in grams. (It does not matter if the egg was stored for a day or two prior to incubation - its weight loss during this period will not normally have been great enough to make a significant difference).

2. Find the "Initial Weight" on the chart which is closest to your egg weight.

3. Re-weigh the egg after 1 or 2 days' incubation, and again after 3 or 4 days' incubation. It is important that the egg be weighed at the same time each day, so that the intervals between the weighings will be consistent.

4. Figure out what the daily weight loss has been and compare it with the appropriate figures on the chart. If it seems within limits, the egg will usually not need to be weighed again until just before hatching, to confirm the earlier findings. Generally, an egg that starts off on a certain percentage weight loss line will continue losing weight at that same rate, provided the incubation conditions stay the same.

5. If weight loss seems a lot greater or a lot less than what it should be, check first of all that your calculations are correct. If there is any doubt, re-weigh at the same time the following day to confirm your suspicions. Once a problem is confirmed, take the appropriate steps (as outlined previously in the text) to

Table 10.6 - Egg Weight Loss Chart

INITIAL WEIGHT	TARGET WT. LOSS: 13%		TARGET WT. LOSS: 15%		TARGET WT. LOSS: 17%	
OF EGG	DAILY LOSS	FINAL WT.	DAILY LOSS	FINAL WT.	DAILY LOSS	FINAL WT.
370	0.96	322	1.11	314	1.26	307
375	0.97	326	1.12	319	1.27	311
380	0.99	331	1.14	323	1.29	315
385	1.00	335	1.15	327	1.31	320
390	1.01	339	1.17	331	1.33	324
395	1.03	344	1.18	336	1.34	328
400	1.04	348	1.20	340	1.36	332
405	1.05	352	1.21	344	1.38	336
410	1.07	357	1.23	348	1.39	340
415	1.08	361	1.24	353	1.41	344
420	1.09	365	1.26	357	1.43	349
425	1.10	370	1.27	361	1.44	353
430	1.12	374	1.29	365	1.46	357
435	1.13	378	1.30	370	1.48	361
440	1.14	383	1.32	374	1.50	365
445	1.16	387	1.33	378	1.51	369
450	1.17	391	1.35	382	1.53	373
455	1.18	396	1.36	387	1.55	378
460	1.20	400	1.38	391	1.56	382
465	1.21	405	1.39	395	1.58	386
470	1.22	409	1.41	399	1.60	390
475	1.23	413	1.42	404	1.61	394
480	1.25	418	1.44	408	1.63	398
485	1.26	422	1.45	412	1.65	403
490	1.27	426	1.47	416	1.67	407
495	1.29	431	1.48	421	1.68	411
500	1.30	435	1.50	425	1.70	415
505	1.31	439	1.51	429	1.72	419
510	1.33	444	1.53	433	1.73	423
515	1.34	448	1.54	438	1.75	427
520	1.35	452	1.56	442	1.77	432
525	1.36	457	1.57	446	1.78	436
530	1.38	461	1.59	450	1.80	440
535	1.39	465	1.60	455	1.82	444
540	1.40	470	1.62	459	1.84	448
545	1.42	474	1.63	463	1.85	452
550	1.43	478	1.65	467	1.87	456
555	1.44	483	1.66	472	1.89	461
560	1.46	487	1.68	476	1.90	465
565	1.47	492	1.69	480	1.92	469
570	1.48	496	1.71	484	1.94	473
575	1.49	500	1.72	489	1.95	477
580	1.51	505	1.74	493	1.97	481
585	1.52	509	1.75	497	1.99	486
590	1.53	513	1.77	501	2.01	490
595	1.55	518	1.78	506	2.02	494
600	1.56	522	1.80	510	2.04	498
605	1.57	526	1.81	514	2.06	502
610	1.59	531	1.83	518	2.07	506
615	1.60	535	1.84	523	2.09	510
620	1.61	539	1.86	527	2.11	515
625	1.62	544	1.87	531	2.12	519
630	1.64	548	1.89	535	2.14	523
635	1.65	552	1.90	540	2.16	527
640	1.66	557	1.92	544	2.18	531
645	1.68	561	1.93	548	2.19	535
650	1.69	565	1.95	552	2.21	539
655	1.70	570	1.96	557	2.23	544
660	1.72	574	1.98	561	2.24	548
665	1.73	579	1.99	565	2.26	552
670	1.74	583	2.01	569	2.28	556
675	1.75	587	2.02	574	2.29	560
680	1.77	592	2.04	578	2.31	564
685	1.78	596	2.05	582	2.33	569
690	1.79	600	2.07	586	2.35	573
695	1.81	605	2.08	591	2.36	577
700	1.82	609	2.10	595	2.38	581
705	1.83	613	2.11	599	2.40	585
710	1.85	618	2.13	603	2.41	589
715	1.86	622	2.14	608	2.43	593
720	1.87	626	2.16	612	2.45	598
725	1.88	631	2.17	616	2.46	602
730	1.90	635	2.19	620	2.48	606
735	1.91	639	2.20	625	2.50	610
740	1.92	644	2.22	629	2.52	614
745	1.94	648	2.23	633	2.53	618
750	1.95	652	2.25	637	2.55	622

increase or decrease weight loss as needed.

Example 1:

Initial weight of an egg is 433g. It is weighed after 2 days of incubation and again after 5 days of incubation. Its weight after 2 days is 430.6g. After 5 days the weight is 427g. Is it losing weight adequately?

Weight loss after 2 days = $\frac{(433 - 430.6)}{2} = \frac{2.4}{2}$ = 1.2 g DAILY weight loss

Weight loss after 5 days = $\frac{(433 - 427)}{5} = \frac{6}{5}$ = 1.2 g DAILY weight loss

The egg is therefore losing weight at a constant rate, as it should, since the conditions of incubation have been constant. (Significant fluctuations in weight loss rates of eggs could mean there are temperature/humidity fluctuations within the incubator, which should definitely be checked and corrected.)

To see if this weight loss rate falls within the normal parameters, find the initial weight on the chart which is closest to 433 g. It is 435g. At 13% target weight loss, daily loss is 1.13g. At 15%, it is 1.30g. The rate at which this egg is actually losing weight is 1.2 g/day, which falls between these values and is therefore around a 14% weight loss rate. This is well within normal parameters, so no adjustments will be necessary.

Example 2:

Initial weight of an egg is 567g. It is weighed after 9 days of incubation, and its weight at this time is 541.3g. Is weight loss within normal parameters?

Weight loss after 9 days = $\frac{(567 - 541.3)}{9} = \frac{25.7}{9}$ = 2.86g DAILY loss

On the chart, the initial weight closest to 567g is 565g. At the highest weight loss rate on the chart (17%) the daily weight loss is only 1.92 g. The egg's weight loss appears dangerously high;

after 50 days it will have lost a total of (50 x 2.86) = 143 g.

Expressed as a percentage of the original weight, this is:

$$\frac{143}{567} \times 100 = 25.2\ \%$$

Since a 25% weight loss is unacceptably high (death usually occurs at weight loss rates over 20%), adjustments to slow down rate of evaporation must immediately be made in order to save the developing chick. Note, however, that some damage may already have been done, since the egg has already been incubating for 9 days at this high weight loss. The earlier a problem can be caught and corrected, the better the chick's chance for survival, as outlined earlier.

Note that it does an egg no harm to be out of the incubator for a few minutes in order to be weighed. A similar slight cooling is experienced when the male emu gets off his nest in the wild in order to stretch his legs.

10.6 "CSS"- A METHOD FOR ESTIMATING INITIAL WEIGHTS OF EMU EGGS

Monitoring the rate of weight loss in emu eggs because so much individual variation is possible, has proved a very useful tool to many emu farmers, as outlined in **Section 10.5**. Many farmers who have incubated successfully without the use of a scale may decide to purchase one when problems start to occur with the hatch. By the time this decision is made, there may already be many eggs in the incubator. Although weight loss in these eggs can be monitored from that point on, this may be frustrating because without knowing what the initial weight of the egg was, it is hard to know what daily weight loss rate to aim for (as shown in the Egg Weight Loss Chart, **Table 10.6**).

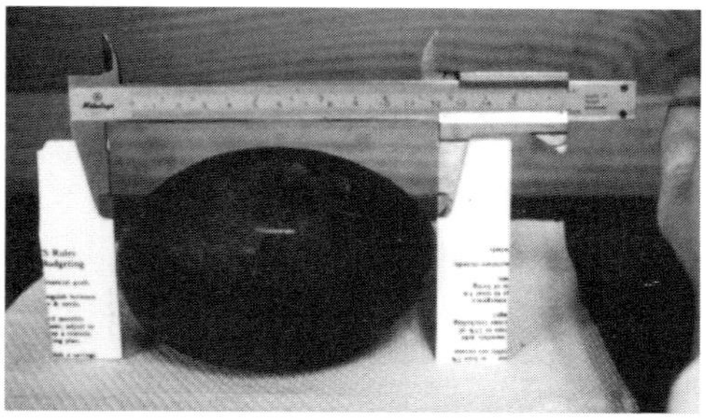

Plate 10.2(a) - Linear measurement of **length** of egg.

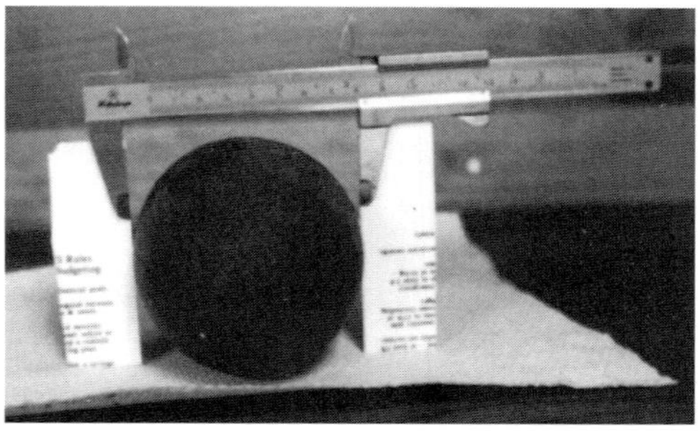

Plate 10.2(b) - Linear measurement of **breadth** of egg.

A method to estimate with reasonable accuracy what the initial weight of the egg was, would be extremely useful in these cases. Thanks to some excellent work done by Hoyt (1979), there is such a method.

According to Hoyt's method, the linear measurements of the egg are used, together with a **coefficient** which varies from species to species, to estimate the initial weight of the egg. These figures are applied to an equation which he devised, in order to calculate initial weight.

The only equipment needed is a good Vernier caliper or some other type of adjustable set square/caliper. **Plate 10.2(a) and (b)** shows how to measure the egg, i.e. **not** along its curvature. The measurement needs to be in millimeters, to give the freshly laid weight in grams.

Provided the "CSS" (Coefficient, Species Specific) for the species of bird is known - in this case, the Emu - , these figures can now be applied to Hoyt's equation. This method works for all bird eggs.

Hoyt's equation is very simple:

W = CSS x L x B x B

where **W** = freshly laid weight of the egg

L = linear measurement of length of egg

B = linear measurement of breadth (width) of egg

CSS = Coefficient for bird species concerned.

However, what is the CSS for emus? Until now, as far as we know, it has not been documented - but after weighing and measuring over 100 fresh emu eggs from 11 different pairs of birds of various ages and applying these figures to Hoyt's equation, with CSS being the only unknown, we have come up with a figure of **0.00056** as the CSS for emus.

Provided the egg is measured accurately, by applying this formula with the CSS of 0.00056, the estimation of the initial egg weight should be accurate to within 10 grams.

Example: An egg which has been in the incubator for 15 days was not initially weighed. Its length is 133.3mm, and its breadth 86.1mm, as measured with a Vernier caliper (see **Plates 10.2(a) and (b)**). What was its initial weight?

W = CSS x L x B x B

W = 0.00056 x 133.3 x 86.1 x 86.1

W = 553g

It should always be remembered that this figure is an estimate only, so that you will have a "beginning figure" to work from which will be reasonably close. The ideal is of course to weigh eggs prior to incubation.

Knowing the CSS of emu eggs, and how to apply it, is also a particularly valuable tool for incubator technicians whose clients are having problems with their hatch. If the incubator company's technician/consultant will take the time and trouble to learn to measure eggs accurately, he can then at least ascertain if humidity levels in the incubator are the cause of the problem or not, based on egg weight loss - even if the eggs have never been weighed before. All the technician needs is an accurate scale, good set of calipers and the formula. While of course this formula cannot solve all problems, it may be able to shed light on some, and therefore, it is worth knowing.

10.7 ASSISTED HATCH

In discussing assisted hatch, it should be remembered that emu egg incubation is still very much at a research stage. As more knowledge and better techniques become available, assistance should become less necessary. At the commercial level, assisting the hatching chick may not be economically feasible.

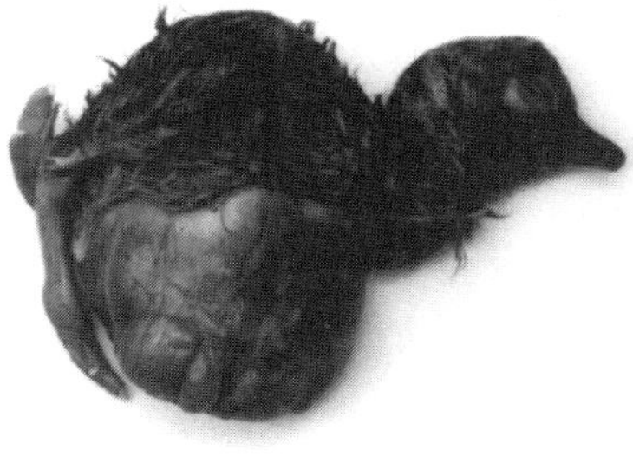

Plate 10.3 - Very unusual malposition - (dead) chick was lying crosswise in egg.

Figs. 10.3 (a) and (b) - Differences in position between correctly positioned and malpositioned ("breech") emu chick.

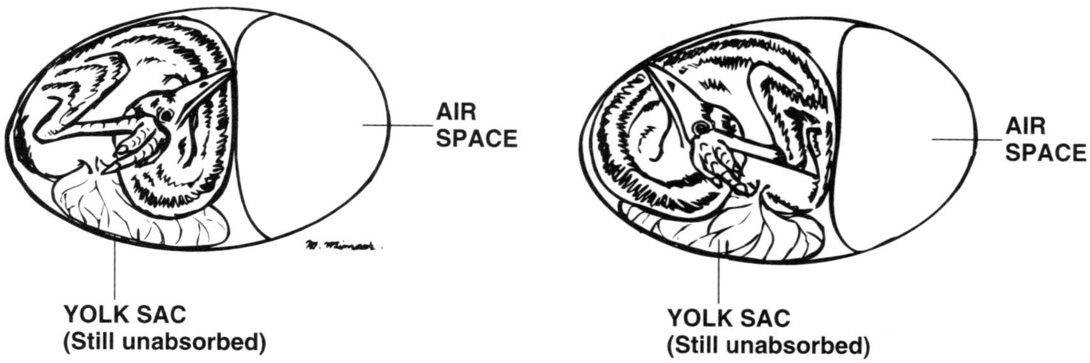

Fig. 10.3(a) - Correctly positioned chick. (a few days prior to hatching).

Fig. 10.3(b) - Malpositioned chick. (soon due to hatch).

(a) CHICK MALPOSITIONING

Some strange malpositions are sometimes seen in emu eggs, such as the very unusual one shown in **Plate 10.3**. Often the causes are unknown. A few malpositions may be related to egg shape and/or egg positioning, as discussed in **Section 9.3.** Torpedo-(football-) shaped eggs seem particularly prone to the type of malposition where the chick is turned completely backwards in the egg, i.e. with tail in airspace side, head at other end. (**Fig 10.3(b)**). Eggs which experience insufficient weight loss or have some other problem often contain a malpositioned chick. In these cases, malpositioning is probably a symptom of the problem rather than the problem itself.

An egg should be marked as having a potential for malpositioning if the history of the breeder birds shows more than 3 eggs with the same type of malpositioning in one season. Football-shaped eggs should be watched for this problem as a matter of course.

If most chicks from the "problem" breeder pair are strong and healthy, a large incidence of malpositioning in eggs should not be a reason to cull this pair of birds out of the breeding program. There may be some simple way in which the problem can be lessened or alleviated, and it would be a pity to decide prematurely that the problem was due to "bad genetics" when a simple change in some aspect of the management of such birds could cure the problem.

If malpositioning is suspected due to one of the above reasons, or simply because the egg is due/overdue, feels hot to the touch and moves a little when set on counter - but has not sounded properly - the egg may be opened by cracking a small hole in the airspace end of the egg. This end will still be felt as the cooler end, since the chick has not succeeded in breaking through. After washing hands, dip finger in some clean water, insert finger through the hole made in the egg and gently dampen the membrane. There will be a fairly large airspace and the membrane will generally be white and follow the contours of the chick. Wet down all of the visible inner membrane. This will cause it to become quite transparent. Look for two things:

1. **The chick's beak** - if it cannot be seen but is in the right position after all, its point can be easily felt and will be distinguishable from any other part of its anatomy. Slight pressure on the beak should cause it to push back, sometimes with a slight pecking motion. If the beak is found, the chick is not malpositioned and the hole may be taped over to let the chick hatch in his own good time.

2. **Blood vessels (red) in the membrane** - This is usually an indication that the chick is not yet ready to hatch, since the blood supply in the chorio-allantois (just under the inner shell membrane) is still active. If there are no red blood vessels but only brown ones, and the chick's body can be seen quite well under the transparent membrane, the chick should be ready to hatch, and little or no bleeding will occur if the membrane is torn. Therefore it should be safe to open the egg further, with due care of course.

If no beak is felt, there may be one or two round protrusions that can be felt through the membrane and which are the bird's hocks. This means the chick is breech. Even if there is some blood in the membrane, intervention will be necessary at this stage. However, in order to minimize bleeding which could cause harm to the chick, the airspace end is taped shut without breaking through any membranes and an effort is made to locate the bird's head on the other side. Roll the egg on a flat surface to let it come to rest in the correct position. Then, based on the normal hatching position, estimate where the chick's head is - perhaps an inch from the apex of the egg, non-airspace end, and down the side a little. Make a small hole in the egg and gently peel away the shell and outer (white) membrane attached to the shell. The inner (white) membrane should be visible; or else, if you have found the right spot, there will be an area of brownish discoloration. This is where the chick's beak is trying to penetrate. Remove enough shell and membrane to expose the beak, and leave him to hatch on his own if possible. This should now be less of a problem since he is no longer in danger of suffocation. Note: a brown spot in the membrane, whether in a correctly positioned or malpositioned chick, means that the blood supply has been withdrawn from that area and the membrane will not bleed there if torn.

In attempting to locate a chick's beak, several places on the egg may need to be cracked and some bleeding in membranes may occur. Try to stop any bleeding by use of pressure and Betadine solution, and tape over any holes that were in the wrong place. Occasionally a chick's head is found tucked under him between his legs. This is a position too awkward to hatch from, so more human assistance than usual will be needed if you are fortunate enough to find such a chick still alive.

Note that some malpositioned chicks may not have absorbed their yolk sacs completely, so as much time in the egg as possible should be given them in order to do so. If no progress is made in about 2 days (use your judgment), further hatching assistance should be given, a little at a time.

On occasion, a malpositioned chick will actually succeed in breaking through the inner shell membrane. Faint cheeping may then be heard, and it is essential that the chick's beak be found and exposed as soon as possible, or he will probably suffocate. The egg may start to "sound" at this point, but perhaps not as definitely as in a normal egg. Some chicks are actually strong enough to hatch out of the wrong end of the egg completely unassisted.

(b) THE EGG WITH EXCESSIVE WEIGHT LOSS

An egg that is discovered to have lost around 20% of its original weight already on its 43rd or 44th day of incubation, but is still alive (jiggling), can sometimes be saved by some intervention:

1. Open a hole in the airspace end of the egg, but do not tear the inner membrane.

2. The airspace will be larger than normal, and the white inner membrane may look almost "sucked-down" over the chick. Wet the membrane as described previously in **Section 10.7(a)**. Blood vessels will still be very red and prominent in the membrane, but this is good since the idea is to supply the blood vessels with plenty of **air** (by means of the hole in the shell) as well as **water** because the chick is getting dehydrated from the excessive weight loss. It is hoped that the blood vessels can take up some of the water used to wet the membrane and transport it to the chick. The water also gives pliability to the membrane so the chick will not be stuck tight under it and be unable to hatch.

3. Tape a thick piece of absorbent gauze over the hole and wet it thoroughly, to keep inside of egg moist. Re-wet membrane and gauze whenever they start to dry out, at least 3 times a day. Keep doing this for several days, with the egg in the (humid) hatcher, until it becomes due. By now the blood vessels should have turned brownish and the membrane will be more transparent on wetting. The chick's beak should break through the membrane eventually (often a day or so earlier than the "due date") and after that it is no longer necessary to keep wetting down the membrane: the chick should be able to hatch by himself. He will probably be fairly small and will have used up more of his yolk sac than normal, so drinking and eating will need to be encouraged a day or so earlier than usual.

Relationship Between Egg Weight and Chick Weight

A normal, healthy chick will weigh approximately $\frac{2}{3}$ of what the egg weighed initially. 2/3 = 0.66666666 (0.67)

$$\text{i.e.}\quad \frac{\text{chick weight}}{\text{initial egg weight}} = 0.67$$

If egg weight loss was higher than normal during incubation, the chick will weigh less than it ought to and therefore the figure will be lower, e.g. 0.61 or even as low as 0.56 in a chick that became quite dehydrated.

If egg weight loss was lower than normal, the chick may be a little edematous (bloated or swollen) and/or have a small amount of yolk sac sticking out on hatching, which can be gently pushed inside after generous lubrication with antiseptic ointment. The figure will then be higher, e.g. 0.69 or even 0.71.

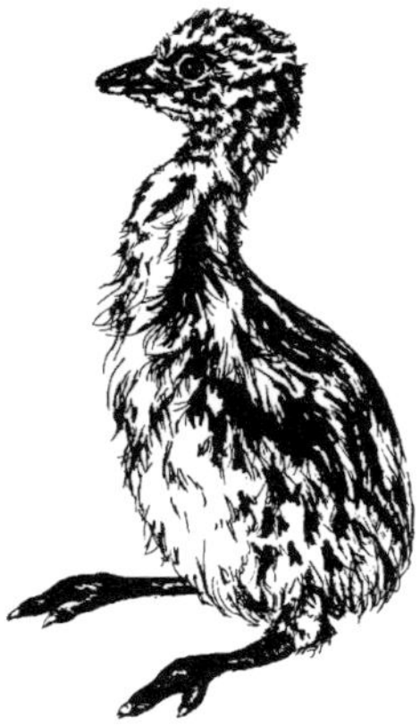

Some chick problems can be traced back to insufficient or excessive weight loss during incubation. "Head-weaving", for instance, often occurs in chicks with egg weight losses close to 20%. It does not appear to do lasting damage, however. It may be due to a fluid imbalance or possibly thiamin deficiency (see **Section 6.4(b)**).

10.8 EGGS THAT FAIL TO HATCH

Whenever possible, eggs that go over their due date and fail to hatch should be opened to try to determine what the problem was. Some answers may not be apparent right away, but if all information is faithfully recorded, the reading of one's notes two or three years down the line may suddenly give an answer to what the problem could have been.

If for no other reason, it is important to open eggs in order to determine which eggs are infertile. While there may be a few eggs that look infertile but are not (died soon after fertilization), there will be no mistake about eggs that have some blood development in them, or a visible embryo in addition to blood vessels: these are definitely fertile.

A large number of infertile (or apparently infertile) eggs from any one pair raises the question of whether the pair is still compatible, or whether the male's sperm production is being reduced, perhaps due to some nutritional imbalance or deficiency (see **Section 13.3**.)

A large number of dead embryos again raises the question of whether the breeder diet is adequate: but it also points to the possibility of "pilot error", i.e. some problem in the handling or incubation of the eggs. Perhaps eggs are being overcrowded in a small incubator with inadequate ventilation, and this is causing competition between all eggs for available oxygen.

Another potential problem is failure to check incubator/hatcher settings regularly. Because most emu egg incubation is not done on an "all-in, all-out" basis, but eggs are continually added to an incubator until it is full, one tends to forget that as the embryos grow, not only do they all require increasing amounts of oxygen but they also start to generate more heat. This can push the temperature in the incubator up to an unacceptable level, if the thermostat is not reset. The reverse can happen as more of the eggs are moved to the hatcher. Moreover, any time that a pan of water is allowed to run dry in a small incubator or hatcher, this also tends to push the temperature up. Due to all these variables the incubators must be continuously monitored.

Note that it is difficult to tell the difference simply by looking into eggs between excessively high weight loss and excessively low weight loss as cause of death in eggs, if the embryo has died any time during the first 35 or so days of the incubation period. In either of these eggs there will be an embryo floating around in liquid, because of the stage at which it died. The fact that in one case the liquid is more concentrated and in the other more dilute cannot of course be seen, except in very extreme cases of high weight loss where the egg contents will appear very viscous. Egg weight measurement is the only really accurate way of knowing, although some signs may help one to guess at the problem, such as the airspace end being tilted way up (more than is normal) in the egg with excessively high weight loss. The air space will be correspondingly large.

One further interesting point is the difference in smell between infertile eggs and those which contain a dead embryo or dead chick. The infertile egg, provided it is uncontaminated, will have a rather pleasant, sweet smell. The egg with an embryo in it will not have this distinct smell but may smell faintly similar to a newly hatched chick, if uncontaminated. If infected, of course, either egg will smell "eggy" or bad. This is useful when wishing to preserve eggshells intact for decorating purposes: one can make just a tiny hole in the egg that failed to hatch, smell it, and know which eggs can successfully be blown. All other eggs should be broken open to examine the dead embryo, hopefully to learn something from it. Taking photographs to complement one's notes can be a great help in later diagnosis of a problem and in furthering research.

Even if temperature has been set correctly and weight loss is monitored to ensure correct humidity levels, there are still several additional factors that can cause an embryo to die in the egg. Here are some of them:

- **Unacceptable temperature fluctuations** - (e.g. temperature shoots up above 100°F and remains high for several hours before a faulty thermostat is detected; or there is a power failure and temperature drops to the 70's for several hours.) Prevention: monitor incubators often, and have a small alarm next to your bed that goes off when power is interrupted. Keep a generator on hand in case of extended periods of power failure.

- **Very erratic humidity levels** - This becomes a problem if the incubator does not have automatic humidity control, and is not in a climate-controlled environment. For this reason, keeping the incubator in a barn or outbuilding where the humidity of the air changes according to the weather outside, is not a good idea.

- **Carbon dioxide buildup** - (insufficient air flow). If the levels of carbon dioxide in an incubator become too high because the incubator is filled with eggs that are using more and more oxygen as their embryos grow, and the air is not being vented and replaced with fresh air fast enough, the developing chicks can die from lack of oxygen and/or toxic levels of carbon dioxide. The closer an egg is to hatching, the greater the chick's need for oxygen; therefore levels which were just sufficient to support its growth before are no longer sufficient and the chick dies just prior to hatch. Prevention: do not pack small cabinet-type incubators too full (these are the kind of incubators in which this problem is most frequently seen), keep all vents completely open, keep a ceiling fan on (or fan that blows air past the vent holes of the incubator), and open incubator fairly frequently to allow the entry of fresh air, especially towards the end of incubation.

- **Jarring of eggs** - during handling or turning. Eggs can withstand a certain amount of bumping into each other, since this will happen in the wild when the male shuffles the eggs around in the nest to turn them. Extreme jarring or dropping eggs, e.g. while weighing, can be harmful. In incubators without dividers and containing only a few eggs, the eggs may also roll around and knock into each other more than is desirable, during automatic turning. Prevention: use wire separators or dividers in incubators; turn eggs gently if turning by hand, and handle with care in general.

- **Inadequate or improper turning** - If turning is not done regularly as well as frequently, problems may result. Forgetting to hand turn eggs for several days, or leaving the automatic turner off by mistake, may result in a higher incidence of malpositions or even death in some eggs that are at a critical stage of development when this occurs. Incidence of problems will depend on how long the eggs remained unturned. Generally, the embryo will stick to the shell membranes at the top or the yolk sac will stick to the bottom of the egg, and normal development cannot take place. When hand turning, the egg must not be continuously rotated in one direction, but back and forth, or this could also cause problems.

- **Infection in eggs** - Eggs could become infected, resulting in damage and/or death to the developing embryo, in 4 ways:

  1. FROM INCUBATOR. Harmful fungi (molds), bacteria or viruses may be growing in an incubator that was not properly cleaned and fumigated prior to setting eggs. Harmful organisms may also grow in the water-pan, if there is one. Prevention: clean and fumigate incubator before placing eggs in it, and put a little disinfectant into any water-trays periodically.

  2. FROM THE HEN. Certain diseases can be "vertically transmitted", i.e. pass from hen to developing egg. Prevention: place breeders on broad spectrum antibiotic prior to laying season if problem is suspected. Vaccinate

breeders against any viral diseases known to be a problem in emus in your area. In this way, chicks are hatched temporarily protected against such diseases rather than infected.

3. FROM BEING LAID IN WET/DIRTY ENVIRONMENT. An egg needs to dry as soon as possible after being laid, so that the cuticle (the final, transparent secretion) can dry on the egg and temporarily seal up its pores to protect it from the entry of harmful organisms. As the egg cools, its contents shrink slightly, and if laid in wet and dirty conditions, any bacteria present on the wet egg can easily be sucked in through the pores, which are still open.

4. FROM OTHER INFECTED EGGS. If there is a rotten, oozing egg in the incubator and its contents seep onto other eggs - or worse, explode onto other eggs - the high concentration of harmful bacteria will almost certainly cause some infection problems among the eggs. If a rotten egg does burst, the incubator and eggs should be washed immediately with hot disinfectant solution (must be a product that is safe for eggs - a solution of chlorine bleach will work) and the incubator should preferably be re-fumigated before eggs are replaced. In the meantime, continue to incubate washed eggs in a standby incubator, label them "at-risk" and keep separated from uncontaminated eggs if possible. Prevention: regular checking of incubators for any faint whiff of rotten egg, and removing any smelly eggs promptly.

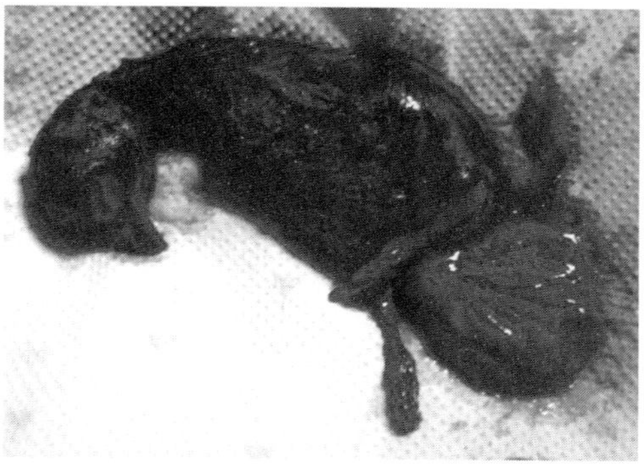

Plate 10.4 (a) - Dead embryo with "parrot beak" and "clubbed-down" feathers on belly - signs of B-vitamin or manganese deficiency in breeders.

- **Nutritional deficiencies in breeder birds**. - Several different types of nutritional deficiencies, notably in the B-vitamins but also some other vitamins and trace elements, can cause embryonic mortality at various stages of incubation. These have been fairly well documented for turkeys and chickens. From this documentation it is possible to make an educated guess as to the causes of certain embryonic abnormalities seen in emu eggs. One interesting and very easily recognizable abnormality is the "parrot beak", caused in poultry by a deficiency either of biotin (a B-vitamin), folacin (also a B-vitamin) or manganese (a trace element). The emu embryo shown in **Plate 10.4(a)** also had "clubbed-down" feathers, caused in poultry embryos by a deficiency in riboflavin (another B-vitamin).

It is quite possible that the laying hen's diet was borderline-deficient in several or all of these nutrients, and that some additional stress at the time the egg was being produced depleted her even further. The hen in question did not produce any other deformed embryos in that season. However, this shows that in any nutritional deficiency, more than just one factor are usually involved. Along with parrot-beak, another general sign of breeder deficiency of several of the B-vitamins and manganese, is dwarfing and shortening of leg bones. A most interesting living example of all these signs is seen in **Plate 10.4(b)**. This bird came from breeders located several hundred miles from the embryo shown in **Plate 10.4(a)**.

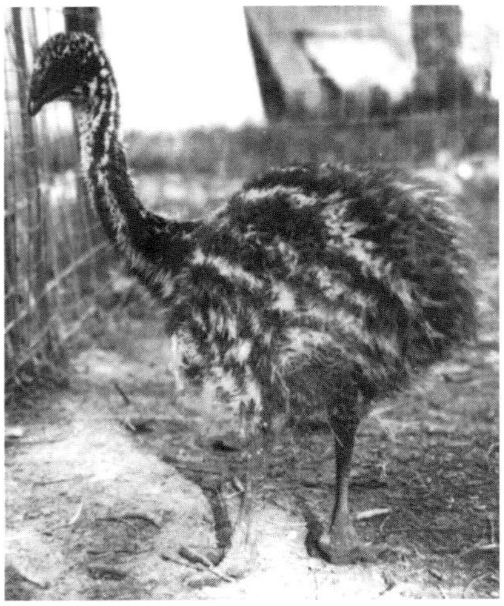

Plate 10.4(b) - A rare example of "parrot beak" in a living chick.

Problems involving dead embryos do not always have a straightforward answer, as can be seen from the text. Suspected infections in eggs/embryos can of course be cultured by the closest avian diagnostic laboratory, starting with tests for the most common poultry diseases known in the area. Some diseases are only transmitted in specific ways, and so, once a harmful organism has been positively identified as the cause of a problem, steps for prevention of the problem in the future as well as for a cure can be taken.

Overall, prevention is better than cure. By maintaining a good nutritional program, providing clean sheltered laying areas and incubating eggs properly, most problems can be avoided and good production will result.

10.9 POST-HATCH CHICK PROBLEMS/CHICK DEATHS

In gathering data from many different breeders, there were many cases of chick losses soon after hatch. These could generally be related to incorrect conditions of incubation, as follows:

INCUBATOR CONDITIONS	**CHICK CONDITION**
Temperature too low.	Weak chick taking longer to hatch, needing assistance
Temperature too low and humidity too high, or fluctuating greatly.	Weak, swollen chick (edematous), mushy looking, needing hatching assistance. Sometimes a dirty green stool is passed in the egg just prior to hatching. Higher incidence of chick malpositions.
Temperature too low, humidity too high or fluctuating, and too little oxygen (poor airflow due to poor incubator). Also possible buildup of carbon dioxide to toxic levels.	Any of the above, plus blotchy beak and legs, yolk sac sometimes not fully absorbed or not absorbed at all, red around eyes and legs, deformities. Survivors would often have higher incidence of retained yolk sac problems and leg problems later on.

INCUBATOR CONDITIONS *(cont.)*	**CHICK CONDITION**
Temperature too high.	Premature hatching of chicks, sometimes before yolk sac has had time to be absorbed properly. Again, survivors may have retained yolk sac problems and/or leg problems.

N.B. An excessively high temperature in the hatcher, especially if aggravated by poor airflow, can also cause death to hatching chicks through overheating and suffocation. As can be seen from this very general list, there is always a danger in extremes. In incubation as in nutrition and many other life processes, the thing to strive for is the correct balance of factors.

10.10 THE YOLK SAC

Role of the Yolk Sac

The part of an egg known as the "yolk sac" deserves special discussion due to its importance to the proper growth and development of the chick. In an infertile egg, of course, the yolk sac does not undergo any changes and remains just a plain yolk. When an egg is fertilized, however, a small germinating area on the yolk surface known as the blastodisc, begins to grow and will eventually, given the right conditions, become a chick. This means that the fertilized egg must, when laid, already contain all the necessary nutrients for the complete growth and development of the embryo into a chick. The role of the yolk sac is to provide the majority of these nutrients. In fact, it will keep providing the chick with food for several days after hatching as well, as described under "Absorption of the Yolk Sac".

The Embryo and the Yolk Sac

After just a few days of incubation, the embryo is recognizable as a chick. Resembling a small pink piece of flesh, it has the rudiments of a beak; two large dark protruding areas where the eyes are forming; a long spaghetti-like neck and a tiny body attached in its middle (navel area) to the comparatively large yolk sac. A rudimentary gut is beginning to grow at the point of this attachment, and as the chick grows and its intestinal system develops inside its body, its small intestine will

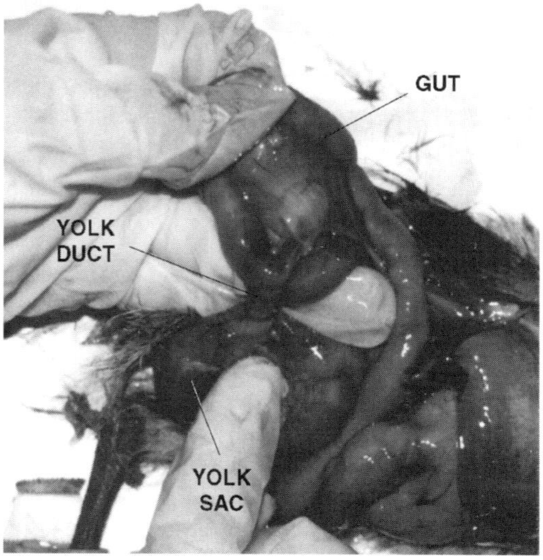

Plate 10.5 - Photograph showing open yolk duct between yolk sac and gut, making it possible to push yolk contents into gut.

remain connected to the yolk sac on the outside by means of a short tube (the yolk duct) passing through the navel opening. A network of blood vessels also grows from the embryo to eventually cover the whole surface of the yolk sac. According to some textbooks dealing with poultry, this network of blood vessels is the only means by which nutrients are carried from the yolk to the chick. However, our opinion is that yolk material can and does also pass directly into the gut of the developing chick and that absorption occurs in this way as well, since in dissections of dead chicks, plenty of yolk material can be found in the gut. It may be a lime-green to dark green color due to the infusion of bile to aid digestion.

Recognizing the Yolk Sac

On opening an egg that has failed to hatch and finding a dead chick, it is usually not difficult to recognize the yolk sac as it will probably still be partially or completely outside of the chick's body. It is a large flaccid sac, at least as large as the chick's body in most cases, and is still attached to the chick via the navel opening. It is often lobed, and is covered with a network of blood vessels interlaced over its surface. Its color may vary between yellow and dirty green. Green areas in parts of the yolk sac are not necessarily a sign of infection; the discoloration may be due to the influx of bile from the chick's gut. The yolk sac walls are quite thin, and it is possible for a chick's toenail to rupture it, although this is not a common occurrence.

Absorption of the Yolk Sac

The contents of the yolk sac are not all used up by the end of an egg's incubation period, nor are they intended to be. There must be enough nutrients left in the yolk sac, on hatching, to provide the chick with everything he needs for at least the first two or three days of his life. This is the crucial time in which an emu chick in the wild must learn to forage for his own food by following the example of his father (and of the other chicks hatched), and since food may not always be close at hand, he must have sufficient energy reserves to be able to walk miles, if necessary, at the tender age of one or two days old. Of course, it would hardly be feasible to walk miles dragging a delicate, thin-walled yolk sac under one's belly - so in accordance with the perfect design of nature, the yolk sac is actually drawn up into the chick's body, through the fairly wide navel opening, a day or so prior to hatching. When this process is complete, a thick band of tissue constricts around the navel opening to close it off completely, preventing entry of any bacteria into the chick's stomach cavity. Usually, this process will be complete before the chick finishes breaking out of its shell. The appearance of the navel should be like a deep dimple with a slightly raised ridge around it.

Sometimes, the indrawing or absorption of the yolk sac will have been only just completed by the time the chick hatches, in which case the navel may not be completely closed. In such cases it is important to keep the navel area clean and disinfected, e.g. with a generous amount of Betadine ointment, until the navel has closed. This should prevent the entry of any harmful bacteria.

Unabsorbed Yolk Sac

There are certain conditions that result in a chick hatching with its yolk sac completely or partially unabsorbed - that is, a portion of it is still outside the body on hatching, or worse, the whole sac is dragging about behind it as it tries to move around in the hatcher. This is a very serious situation, and chances for survival are not good for a number of reasons. Firstly, the yolk sac may rupture very easily, causing shock to the chick at the sudden huge loss of what is still its own body fluids. (Tying off the yolk sac or removing it surgically may constitute the same kind of shock, remembering that the network of blood vessels around the sac is also still part of the chick's own blood supply). Secondly, there is danger in the fact that the yolk sac is still attached to the chick's intestine, and if it is being dragged about behind a fairly active chick, this may actually start to pull some of the chick's intestines out of its body via the navel opening. Finally, since the yolk sac ought to be inside the chick's body by now, there is obviously an underlying problem causing the yolk sac to be unabsorbed, and to achieve success with future hatching, the problem must be found and resolved.

If, however, only a portion of the yolk sac is out, it may be possible to lubricate the area with a disinfectant ointment and gently push the remnant in through the navel opening. The area may be covered with plastic wrap (generously smeared with the same ointment) to keep it supple and lubricated, increasing chances for absorption and proper closure of the navel. The wrap may be held in place by a bandage wrapped firmly around the chick's body and fastened with tape. The chick is usually kept in the hatcher an extra day or two, until the process is complete.

However, if there is more yolk sac out than about the size of a small apricot, chances of survival are greatly reduced. While one may have to accept the loss of a chick in such a case, it is important to look into the possible reasons for the problem - especially if several such cases occur in a row - so that this can be prevented in the future. Here are some possible reasons:

1. **Wet/infected eggs** - if eggs were laid under very wet and muddy conditions, they may have become infected. This could mean bacteria are actually growing in the yolk sac, and the chick will be very weak and sick.

2. **"Helping" the egg hatch** - An over-anxious emu farmer, thinking an egg is overdue, may break into it too soon and too aggressively, before the yolk sac absorption process has been completed. While the decision to break into an egg is justified in some cases, there is a way to go about it that will not harm the chick unduly if he is not due. See **Section 10.7**.

3. **Humidity too high** - if the egg has not lost the appropriate amount of moisture, the chick will be swollen and edematous, the air space smaller than it should be and the yolk sac bigger than it ought to be since it still contains more water than it should. To squeeze this larger-than-normal yolk sac into the more-bloated-than-normal chick is a feat that cannot always be accomplished.

4. **Lack of oxygen** - in an incubator with insufficient air flow, there may not be enough oxygen for the normal process of respiration by the chick - i.e. using up oxygen and food in order to produce energy. Less oxygen available would mean less food (from yolk sac) is used up, so the yolk sac may be larger than normal at hatch and cannot be absorbed properly.

5. **Other factors** - Any problems with the incubator - such as temperature/humidity fluctuations, poor air flow, repeated power failures or a combination of these things, could lead to many problems at hatching including unabsorbed yolk sac.

Retained Yolk Sac

Retained yolk sac is a chick problem which differs from unabsorbed yolk sac in that the yolk sac has been completely drawn into the chick's body just prior to hatching - but its contents fail to be utilized, resulting in a chick with the following symptoms:

1. **Fat belly** - the belly is tight and distended and does not become soft, as it should after two or three days at the very latest. Little or no dark green stool is passed.

2. **Waddling gait** - chick walks like a duck because of the distended belly; may have trouble getting his legs under him at all.

3. **Failure to grow** - although the chick may succeed in eating a little, the presence of the enormous yolk sac in his abdomen not only makes him feel full but also leaves very little space for the intake of food into the gut.

4. **Dry, dull feathers** - again, as a result of malnutrition. The chick is getting very little food either by eating or from his yolk sac.

5. **Shrivelled, skinny legs and emaciation** - due to inadequate intake of both food and water; moreover, the retained yolk sac will often begin to cause a fluid imbalance in the chick. It has been suggested that the yolk sac may even by simple osmotic pressure be drawing in fluids from the chick's own system, dehydrating the chick.

6. **Swelling of inner eyelid/eyelids gummed together** - again, from dehydration.

7. **Wheezy chirp** - fluid imbalances could be causing the entry of water into lungs or air sacs, or possibly it is the pressure of the yolk sac itself causing prob-

lems, as it occupies such a large area of the chick's body. Sometimes "clicking" sounds are also heard as the chick breathes.

8. **Splayed-out leg, curled-in toes or other growth abnormalities** - these are secondary characteristics, caused by deficiencies as a result of malnutrition.

9. **Death** - chick usually dies anywhere between the age of 3 days to 3 weeks. Post-mortem examination will confirm the diagnosis: yolk sac is huge, tube between yolk sac and gut completely or almost completely closed off; chick is emaciated. (In a normal 3-week-old chick, the yolk sac should only be the size of a small pea.)

Although some cases of retained yolk sac are due to an infection present, the majority probably are not. Opinions differ as to probable causes, but the majority of cases have occurred in eggs which experienced insufficient weight loss during incubation. Insufficient oxygen also seemed to be a contributing factor.

We believe that in retained yolk sac, the yolk duct connecting yolk sac to small intestine shuts off prematurely. This means that yolk material can no longer pass directly from the yolk sac to the gut. Although the system of blood vessels surrounding the yolk sac can probably help in the uptake of some of its contents, the sheer volume of the yolk sac means that this could take a very long time. Besides, if uptake of nutrients by the blood vessels was the only method by which yolk contents could be utilized, then retained yolk sac would never be a problem.

Our belief that the ability or failure to utilize the contents of the yolk sac is directly dependent on whether the yolk duct has closed or not, is based on the following observations:

- In all chicks that had died from retained yolk sac, post-mortem examination revealed that the yolk duct was completely constricted and yolk material could not be squeezed through.

- On the other hand, normal chicks who had died due to accidents or acute infections had smaller yolk sacs (indicating that the material was being used up) and although the yolk duct in some cases had a visible constricted area, it was still not difficult to squeeze yolk material from yolk sac into gut. Possibly the yolk duct has a sphincter type mechanism to allow yolk contents into gut as needed.

- The gut of newly hatched chicks which died from other causes contained material in the small intestine on either side of the connection with the yolk duct which looked exactly the same as the contents of the yolk sac - a yolky material, greenish due to the infusion of bile which is secreted directly into the small intestine from gall bladder and liver. There was no food material in the upper part of the digestive tract as far as the gizzard and beginning of duodenum. However, the "yolk-type" contents were found continuously from small intestine to large intestine as far as the vent. A darker green color of the material in the large intestine indicates the absorption of water from it.

These observations still do not explain why the yolk duct closes off prematurely. Finding out the answer to that question might, along with good incubation management, help the emu farmer to avoid this problem completely.

It is possible for a veterinarian to do an operation to remove a retained yolk sac. However, the risks and economics of this should always be weighed up first. The bird will need to be anesthetized, which in itself is always a risk, (especially in such a young chick, who is often not in good condition) and will need some good nursing for the first few days after the operation. It will probably be more susceptible to disease, since any maternal antibodies present in the yolk sac for its protection are now gone; it also does not have that reserve of perfectly balanced nutrients afforded by the yolk sac, and may develop deficiencies as a result, even on a fairly adequate diet. The most common deficiency symptom seen is splayed leg, and this usually grows progressively worse. Prevention of the problem by careful monitoring during incubation seems by far the better alternative.

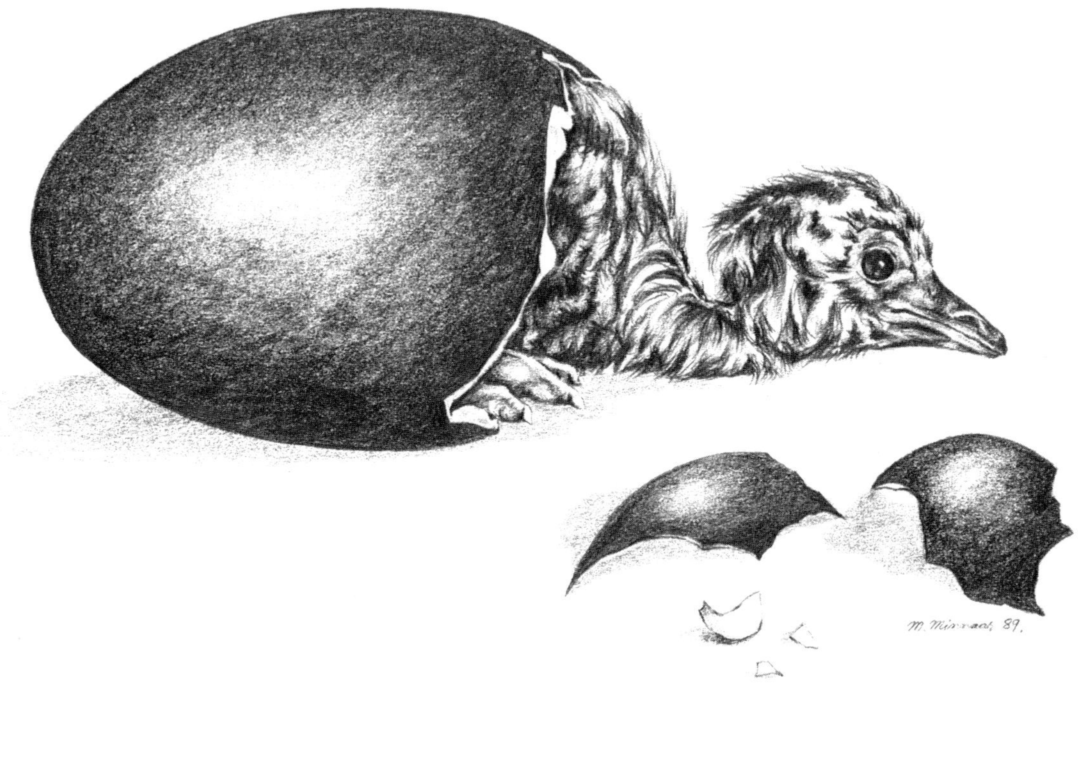

CHAPTER 11

Chick Care

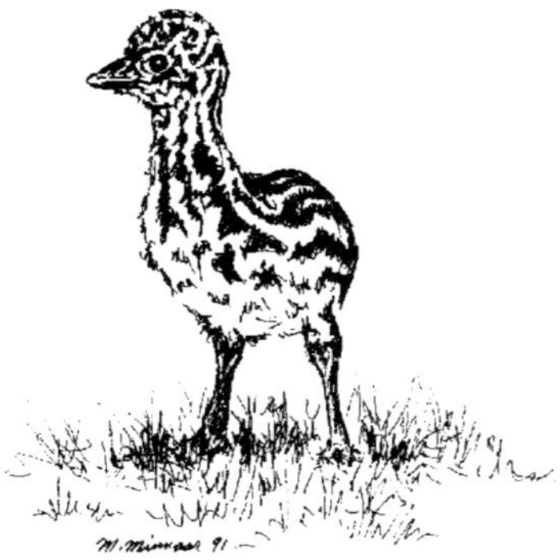

11.1 GENERAL

The needs of a newly hatched emu chick are basically the same as any young animal: proper food, water, warmth, security, sunshine and exercise. Because the yolk sac already provides adequate food for the first few days of its life, warmth and security are the first needs that need to be met. Cleanliness is also very important.

It should be remembered that chick care actually starts with care of the breeders, since a hen on a poor diet cannot put into the egg what she lacks in her own body. Chick care continues with incubation, since any stresses experienced by the egg will naturally affect the developing embryo within. When the chick hatches, direct chick care begins. Even the most excellent chick care, however, is not always enough to counter the effects of poor breeder nutrition or improper incubation. Also, the genetic makeup of a chick (inherited from the parents) may mean that its growth rate or its ability to absorb certain nutrients from its feed is different from the others. All these factors mean that there will be some variations among chicks even though they are raised in exactly the same way. It would not be wise to make any drastic changes to one's feeding or management program if only one or two chicks show leg deformities or stunting, while all the others are normal and healthy. If a large number of chicks start to develop leg problems, however, some changes should definitely be made once the cause of the problem has been found or guessed at. (See **Chapter 6** on Nutrition).

11.2 IN THE HATCHER

Once a chick has hatched, it can be left in the warm environment of the hatcher for as little as a few hours or as much as two days. The usual time period is about 12 to 24 hours, depending on how active the chick is. Since the wire-mesh trays of a hatcher may be a little abrasive on the legs of a very active chick, active chicks with a navel that is nicely closed and dry are often removed sooner. Another reason for this is that unless some form of tall divider is placed at the back of the hatching tray (such as a stiff piece of cardboard with holes so as not to interrupt air flow too much), the active chick may jump out of the tray and end up on the slippery hatcher floor. This could result in damage to tendons, causing splayed leg later on.

As a safety precaution, the newly hatched chick's navel may be swabbed with iodine/Betadine solution or other antiseptic liquid or ointment, in order to prevent harmful bacteria from entering the chick's body via this route. If the navel is nicely closed, Betadine solution is preferable to the ointment since it will dry quickly. If there is a very small portion of yolk sac sticking out and the navel opening is not quite closed, the ointment is the better to use. The whole area is generously covered with ointment and the end of the yolk sac gently pushed inside the opening so that the ridge of tissue around the navel can close completely over it and seal off the navel. Some massaging may be necessary in order to accomplish this. The ointment helps in that it has a lubricating effect and also ensures that any bacteria will be killed before they have a chance to infect the chick. Within an hour of pushing the yolk sac remnant all the way in, the navel should have closed completely. The chick remains in the hatcher until the navel is properly closed.

Even though the floor of the hatcher is usually wire mesh, the chick may still slip on it to some extent. For this reason, many emu farmers tape the newly hatched chick's legs together at the ankles with masking tape, at a distance about equal to the width of the chick's body so that it can sit properly. The tape may be left on for a day or two, or until the chick starts walking on the ground. Two-to three-day-old chicks can walk with the tape still on since they take very short steps, but after that it generally causes them to trip and fall over, and should be removed. Any splayed-leg problem after the age of 3 days will not benefit from taping anyway, but only cause stress to the bird as he keeps overstepping and falling. Taping is not always necessary, but is recommended for any chick that scrabbles around a lot and seems to have difficulty getting his legs under him. Since the bones are still fairly soft on hatching, taping in such cases will probably be of benefit in preventing damage.

A small, fairly rough-textured towel or cloth is sometimes placed in the hatcher to give the chick better traction without being abrasive. It must of course be clean. Chlorine bleach is an excellent disinfectant for chick towels. If towels/cloths are used, they should not cover the entire hatcher tray but only a portion, so as not to interrupt air flow to the rest of the eggs and hatching chicks.

The hatcher should be kept as clean and free of debris as possible. Egg shells should be promptly removed, and the floor of the hatcher can be wet down with a safe disinfectant and mopped dry with a cloth or paper towels at frequent intervals to prevent the accumulation of too much fluff and debris. Some hatchers have a flat tray in the very bottom which collects all debris and slides out easily for periodic cleaning. The water-pan in the hatcher should also contain a little disinfectant so that it does not become a breeding-ground for bacteria. Cleanliness in the hatcher is especially important if the hatcher is also being used as an incubator for eggs that need higher humidity.

11.3 IN THE "BROODER"

A "brooder" need not be any specialized piece of equipment. The dictionary defines it as "a heated structure used for raising young fowl." It can be as simple as a cardboard box with hay in the bottom and a lamp providing warmth in one corner, or as complex as a three-tiered structure with wire-mesh floors, plexiglass walls and heating from above and below. The reason for having a "brooder" or "brooding area" is simply that during its first week or so of life, the chick is less able to handle extremes in temperature. Therefore the "brooder" must provide a comfortable temperature, and security. It must also be easy to keep clean and be accident-proof, i.e. not have any places where the chick can get its head or legs stuck, injuring or killing itself. Other than that, whatever fits one's individual circumstances, budget and number of birds will work. There should be no more than around 10 chicks to a brooding box or brooding area, and they should be about the same age and size to avoid larger chicks smothering smaller ones while they sleep. Heat lamps should be used with great care, since there is always the danger of killing a chick by overheating or by the lamp falling on him. If small brooder boxes are used, an ordinary light bulb hung over the box will usually provide sufficient warmth. A temperature between 80°F and 90°F is usually comfortable for the young chick, but no matter what the source of heat, there should be enough space to allow the chick to move away from the heat source if it becomes uncomfortably warm. This is even more important when using heat lamps or space heaters. Place a thermometer in the box to be able to check temperature periodically, or feel with the back of the hand.

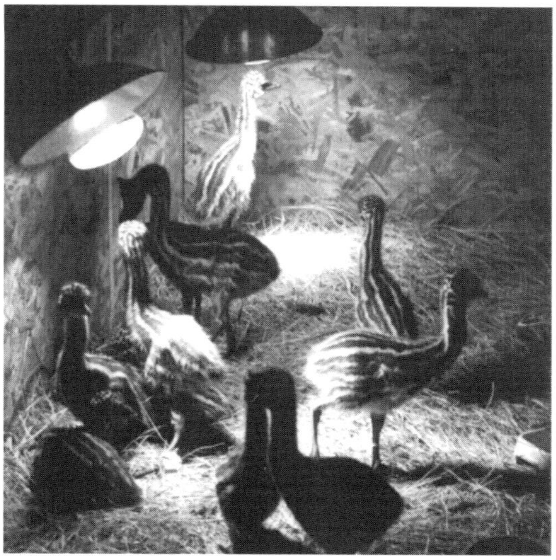

Plate 11.1 - "Brooding Area". An indoor facility for use during cold weather and to sleep small chicks at night.

If the weather is warm and dry, the young chick may be allowed to run outside after only a day in the brooder box or brooding area. As long as the navel is nicely closed, being on the ground will do him no harm and is in fact good for him as he benefits from the sunshine, fresh air and exercise. Curled toes and other minor leg problems seem to straighten out sooner when the chick is allowed out on the ground earlier.

While a small area is sufficient for the first couple of days of life, and will also continue to work as a sleeping area at night, a larger area for daytime exercise is soon needed. Early-hatched chicks which arrive in the middle of winter can obviously not be allowed outside very much (although 10 minutes at a time is not harmful provided it is not raining. For as long as you can stand to be outside bare-footed in cold temperatures, the chick can stand it too.) Therefore an inside run is also needed, both for early-hatched chicks and for inclement weather when chicks are still small. Such facilities are further described in **Section 2.3** ("Chick facilities".)

If chicks chirp incessantly and will not settle down to sleep, check that the temperature in the box is comfortable and not too low (or high). Darkness helps chicks to settle, so if the room is a comfortable temperature and there are at least two chicks together (to share body warmth), the lamp can be switched off for a while and the box covered with a towel to darken it.

11.4 FEEDING THE YOUNG CHICK

Since it derives a lot of nourishment from its yolk sac for the first few days, the chick actually does not need food during this time. On its second day, however, water may be introduced. Using the fact that the chick is attracted to bright colors and contrasts, the chick can be encouraged to drink by floating a few tiny pieces of dark green kale on top of the water, which is in a light-colored dish for better contrast. Stirring the water with the finger or a shiny spoon also encourages the chicks to peck at it. Chick waterers work very well for young emus, provided they cannot be easily tipped over. Once the birds have learned to drink, they seem to enjoy it a lot. It is a good idea to get birds drinking at least 12 hours before offering them food. As a precaution some emu farmers add poultry vitamins/electrolytes (purchased at feed store) to the water for the first few days, to help combat the effects of any "borderline deficiencies" the chicks may have received from the hen.

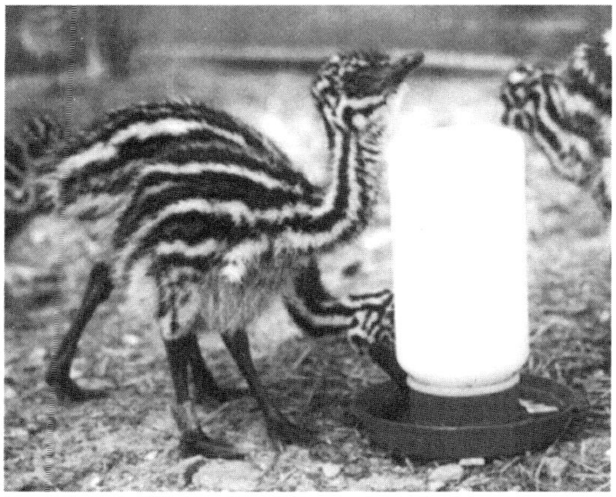

Plate 11.2 - Use of "chick waterers" for young emu chicks.

Feeders and waterers should be tip-proof, as the birds tend to walk in them if at all possible and will spill the feed. This can be accomplished either by using feeders with a very stable base (dog-dish type) or by using off-ground feeders, similar to the kind used in parrot cages where the feeder is hung up against the wall with wire hooks. These feeders can be made from a number of materials, including split PVC piping for a longer feeder.

Many emu farmers start their chicks off with plenty of chopped vegetables such as kale (collard greens), cabbage, spinach, lettuce, carrots and even apples along with some kind of starter crumble. Most fresh feed is eaten with great relish, and by this mixing, the chicks soon learn to eat the starter crumble too. It has been a wise precaution to add plenty of vegetables, since poultry chick starter, turkey starter and gamebird starter have all been possible causes of leg problems in emu chicks, especially if fed free-choice and with no greens or vitamin supplement. Protein levels that were too high along with too-low B-vitamin levels (for emus) may have been a contributing cause. Some ratite starter crumbles have caused the same problems, since the proper diet of the young emu chick has been (and still is) very much a matter of guesswork. Better results have been seen on lower-protein (but high-quality) starter diets, specifically designed for the slower growth of the emu and well fortified with vitamins/minerals.

Starter crumble, chopped greens and in some cases a powdered vitamin/mineral supplement is the standard diet for most emu chicks in their first week of life. "Grit" in the form of small pebbles/bits of gravel should be supplied simultaneously, to help grind up food in the gizzard. Stones and gravel should be freely available in the outside pens. Chicks are usually fed twice a day and food allowed to remain with them for about an hour each time. Feed should not be placed directly under heat lamps, as the heat will "cook away" some of the essential nutrients and will also wilt the greens faster. If chicks are fed inside, there should be sufficient light on the food to stimulate them to eat. Feed may also be stirred with a spoon, pencil or finger to encourage chicks to peck at it. Once one chick is eating, the others generally follow suit eventually.

By the end of the first week, pellets may gradually be introduced into the feed. "Emu grower" or "ratite grower" pellets should ONLY be used on recommendation from other emu farmers who have used it for at least a year and seen no ill effects, since there are many feeds available which are still at the trial-and-error stage. If such pellets are not available, an adequate diet is a 50-50 mixture of 17% poultry lay pellets and rabbit pellets. The rabbit pellets used should be the low-protein (16% or so) kind which contain at least 50% alfalfa, as will be evident by their green color. While this diet may not grow out birds as quickly as some other diets, there are few leg problems on this diet and the birds still reach normal adult size by 12 to 18 months. This diet can be continued up to this time, after which a gradual switch to a breeder pellet is usually recommended, in preparation for the potential first breeding season. If the poultry lay pellet contains a 3:1 or higher ratio of calcium to phosphorus, it would be wise to feed more of the rabbit pellets than the lay pellets to the growing chicks for a better calcium-to-phosphorus ratio. (See **Section 6.5**, "The Balanced Diet"). Alternatively, a little dicalcium phosphate can be sprinkled lightly on the feed every few days, to try to keep the balance more correct.

11.5 OTHER NEEDS

Emus drink a lot from a very early age, especially in hot weather, so fresh water should always be freely available. Large poultry waterers (e.g. 2-to 5-gallon galvanized waterers) or automatic waterers can be used in each pen. Emu droppings are generally very liquid, no doubt partly due to their liking for water, and the farmer should familiarize himself with the normal appearance of the stool so that he will know the difference if a bird actually develops diarrhea. The liquid droppings are usually absorbed very quickly into the ground, so in general very little cleaning of outside pens is necessary, and there is seldom much of a problem with smell. Inside runs, however, will need regular cleaning.

As the chicks get older, they become more robust. Two-to three-month-old chicks rarely need to be closed up at night, except in bad weather. Older chicks are usually given access to a shelter or inside facilities, but are free to roam in and out at will. Most of the time they prefer to sleep outside, in one or two large "huddles" (tight groups) for conserving body warmth. If chicks are shivering or standing hunched-up, they should immediately be moved inside and be given additional warmth (heaters/lamps).

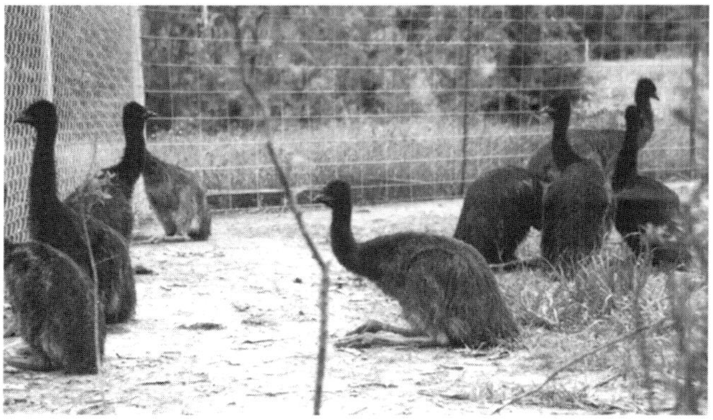

Plate 11.3 - Older chicks in larger outside pens.

Vitamins and electrolytes in the chicks' water is not usually necessary beyond the first few days, if the diet is properly balanced. Some emu farmers never use vitamins/electrolytes; others use it as a safety precaution when the birds have undergone a period of stress, such as chilling, moving or illness. This is a wise idea.

Finally, it is wise to observe the behavior of the birds themselves in order to best care for their needs. Chicks bunching up in a tight huddle are probably cold; chicks chirping loudly and continuously are experiencing some kind of stress; and sluggish, lethargic, panting chicks are probably overheated or sick. Experience will soon help the emu farmer figure out what the chick's behavior is telling him. High humidity along with high temperatures can be very stressful to birds, and since they pant a lot (to lose heat) under these conditions, they will need plenty of fresh water to drink. Putting a sprinkler on for the birds will greatly help alleviate heat stress, and the chicks enjoy wallowing in the water.

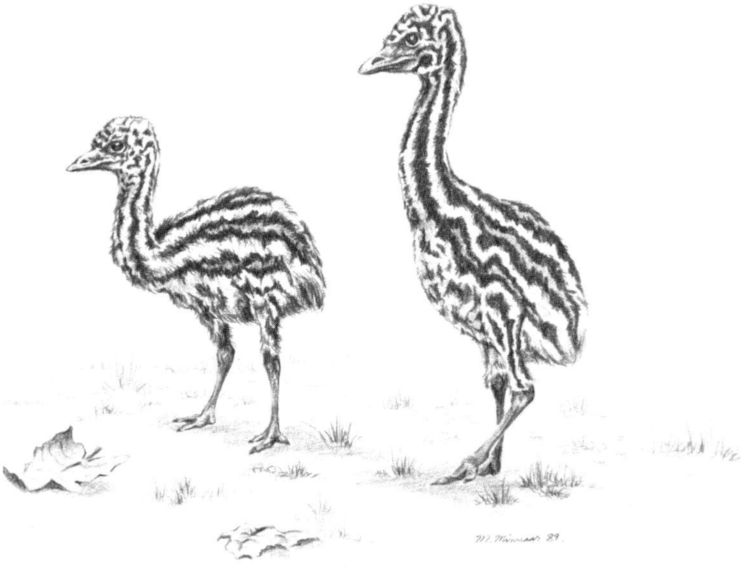

CHAPTER 12

Artificial Insemination of Emus

12.1 POTENTIAL ADVANTAGES OF ARTIFICIAL INSEMINATION

Because emu farming is a relatively new type of livestock industry in America there has only been limited work done on artificial insemination. In the1988/1989 emu breeding season we tried for the first time to inseminate emus using rather primitive methods. Results were not well documented and little follow-up work done, but we did manage to get a few fertile eggs from a hen that was inseminated and had no male with her. Since that time we have worked more on pairing breeders to be compatible than on insemination, but have done considerable work on semen collection. The purpose of this chapter is to make available all our current knowledge and to draw attention to potential problems. A few other individuals with problem emus have used these methods with some success, producing a few live chicks as a result. To date, artificial insemination has mainly been used on hens that are laying eggs but will not accept a mate, fighting and injuring any male with whom they are paired. Obviously the process can only be successful in the breeding season. At other times of the year there will be no ovulation or significant sperm production.

Although some emu hens, particularly seasoned breeders, will lay eggs without the presence of a male, it will be necessary to study just how much influence the male emu has in general on the female as regards the stimulation to begin egg-laying. Artificial insemination of emus, once perfected, could have several advantages:

1. Hens could be fertilized in a more "commercial" way, i.e. could be placed in smaller laying lots during breeding season, saving labor and space and making the operation more efficient.

2. Farmers would not have to contend with fighting and possible injury between birds.

3. Fertility could be greatly increased, particularly in young birds. In other commercial fowl, notably turkeys, artificial insemination has been known to increase fertility by as much as 50%.

4. With time, standards for ideal conformation will be established and the better qualified males could be used a lot more extensively by inseminating. This type of selective breeding, if done correctly, could improve the commercial

species that much sooner.

5. The more inferior males can more readily be culled out of breeding flocks and into feedlots.

6. In turkeys up to 30 eggs can be fertilized with one insemination, making for a labor-efficient process. It is not yet known how many eggs can be fertilized per insemination in emus, and this will certainly affect the feasibility of this process.

12.2 COLLECTING THE SEMEN

The whole artificial insemination process starts with semen collection, then goes on to placing the semen in the oviduct of the hen. While this may sound like a relatively simple process, its success depends largely on the correct handling of both birds and semen, and on the co-operation of the birds. Although it is one of the more scientific parts of emu husbandry, it is still very much an art. With the limited facts available it is important to follow some basic rules and build from experience. There are several points to remember:

1. All birds will not react the same to stimulation, so try to adjust in ways to accommodate the bird.

2. Do not continue trying to collect semen for longer than 10-15 minutes. Rather come back an hour later and try again, to avoid leaving the bird with an aversion for the handling.

3. Always try stimulating freely without restraining the bird. Sometimes this is not possible, but it is still necessary to be as gentle with the bird as possible. If the bird panics, let him go and start again later.

4. Get the job done as quickly as possible.

5. Care should be taken not to allow the semen to be exposed to cold air for too long before placing it in the hen, since this will destroy some of the sperm.

Materials needed are: latex gloves, a plastic collection bag (available from your veterinarian or vet supply store), a sterile syringe (no needle) and a bowl of hot water if it is very cold (to warm the hands in quickly, prior to touching the bird.)

Emu males, if they are tame, will quite readily give semen with a little stimulation. The process of collection is easiest on a voluntary basis and is done basically as follows:

1. Squat down to lower yourself so as not to intimidate the bird. Generally he will approach, strutting back and forth towards you as he recognizes your position as similar to the female breeding position. Exercise patience and he may squat down beside you and start to shuffle towards you on his hocks. Reaching forward to rub the feathers up and down on the front of the bird's neck and chest will often help a more nervous male to squat down. Keep all movements slow but firm.

2. Gently put one forearm against his chest and raise the bird's chest up in front, while he is still in the squatting position. This gets him into proper breeding ("mounting") position.

3. Fairly quickly stimulate the bird with the other hand by pushing firmly against the top of the cloaca if he has not yet exposed his sexual organ (phallus).

4. Once the phallus is exposed, slip the plastic collection bag over it and firmly squeeze the base of the organ (where it joins the body) several times until the bird ejaculates. Then squeeze continuously while he pulls back, until the ejaculation is completed. Still squeezing gently allow the bird to pull out of the bag, thus bringing all the semen out.

5. The male emu will make a shuddering grunting type of sound and his body will be racked with short jerky spasms when he ejaculates. He will also stretch his neck over your shoulder and peck on your back or arm at the same time. If the bird does not do all or some of these things, he generally has not ejaculated and you will not have a semen sample.

Emu males can also be collected under restraint, but with generally poorer results in most cases. This is done as follows:

1. Catch the bird as quickly and quietly as possible. Avoid chasing him around the pen.

2. With someone holding the bird in a standing position, kneel behind him, insert your finger into the cloaca and gently extract the organ. Be very careful in case the bird struggles, not only to avoid injury to the bird but also to yourself. Slip the collection bag over the phallus.

3. Apply the same pressure as in voluntary collection gently but firmly at the base of the organ, so squeezing out any semen already present in the organ. By applying pressure almost as if milking a cow - from base to tip continuously - ejaculation may occur and the collection will yield more semen. The bird's legs may buckle under him when this takes place, so the handler should be ready to support the bird gently until the process is complete, then lower him to the ground.

Wild or nervous birds are generally not very receptive to any form of semen collection and if the bird continually struggles to get away, it is better to abandon further efforts or work on taming the bird first.

If any bleeding occurs around the male organ, cease work on it for a day or two to allow healing, and next time proceed more gently. This may happen in the beginning, but generally the male gets into a routine and no further problems occur. Often on cold days, males may be hard to collect when touched with a cold hand. Try to warm the hand, e.g. in a bowl of hot water, immediately before collection.

The semen of the emu male is normally thick, opaque and a milky white color, but variations do occur where it can be slightly yellowish or more transparent. Occasionally it may appear reddish or orange, which indicates blood in the semen. This is normally the result of rough handling during collection and will usually clear up after a short rest period followed by a few more collections.

Under a microscope the emu semen normally has a very high concentration of spermatozoa per cc. This is common in the avian species. The spermatozoa resemble reptile spermatozoa (e.g. alligator) in shape and length. For the sperm to be effective, good motility should be seen. If semen samples do not resemble this description, e.g. show poor motility, low sperm count or deformed spermatozoa, this could be the result of ineffective collection/handling of the semen, or an unhealthy or immature male, or unsuitable environment for sperm production in the bird. We believe that the male emu needs extended periods of cool environmental temperature in order to produce good sperm. The emu breeding season is in winter both in the northern and southern hemispheres, despite the fact that these occur at opposite times in the year. Although shorter days/longer nights no doubt has an effect on the birds' hormone systems in preparation for breeding and laying, there have been reports (though not yet conclusive evidence) that in unseasonably warm winters or with frequent erratic temperature fluctuations, fertility in eggs has been reduced.

If true, this could mean either that the birds are not breeding as often as they should be, or that the quality or quantity of sperm in the male bird is poorer. Another potential adverse effect on male fertility is obesity. The male emu incubates the eggs in the wild and has a fairly high body temperature. If he is too fat, the testicles may be too well insulated, resulting in poor sperm production.

REASONS TO REJECT SEMEN FOR ARTIFICIAL INSEMINATION

1. If the semen has a low sperm count or contains deformed spermatozoa.
2. If the semen contains feces. Sometimes the male will defecate while a collection is being made and the semen is then unsuitable for use.
3. If there is poor motility or the sperm are dead.
4. If there is other liquid or urates in the semen.

12.3 TREATMENT OF SEMEN

The "sperm" or "spermatozoa" are the living gametes that actually fertilize the eggs of the female. "Semen" refers to the fluid secreted with the sperm as well as the sperm themselves. Sperm need this fluid to exist, and a similar fluid or "extender" can be made and added to the semen of animals in order to dilute it and make the fertilization of more females possible. The number of sperm present is still so great that dilution makes little difference. Extenders are also important as a source of nutrients for the sperm when semen is frozen for later use. The use of specific types of extenders and the possibility of freezing emu semen will still need a lot of research, but in a fresh-cooled (not frozen) emu semen sample, turkey extender has been used and did not seem to have any bad effects on the semen. This sample was not inseminated into a hen but only studied under a microscope.

The normal amount of emu semen collected at a time is about 1cc. This will depend on the male and how co-operative he is. Collections of up to 2cc but also as low as about 0.05cc have been made. The amounts used to inseminate the hen were between 0.2cc and 0.5cc of semen at 7-day intervals. It did not seem to make a difference if less semen was used. The semen was taken straight from the plastic collection bag with a sterile syringe and kept fresh cooled on ice for about 48 hours with no significant change in the quality of the semen. Mostly, however, the fresh semen was placed directly into the hen.

12.4 INSEMINATION OF THE HEN

This part of artificial insemination is less complicated than collection if the hen is co-operative. If the hen can be stimulated quickly and easily with minimal restraint, it is fairly easy to insert the syringe (without a needle) into the oviduct when it is presented. The semen is gently pushed in, the oviduct is released to return into the hen, and the syringe is extracted.

The main factors influencing success in artificially inseminating the hen are:

1. Care to keep the hen from getting over-excited or panicky.
2. The semen must be placed into the oviduct rather than just the cloaca, and in order to do this, the oviduct must be presented by the hen (protruding).
3. Care should be taken when inserting the syringe not to jab the hen in any of this sensitive area, which will cause her to jump up.

As shown in **Plate 12.1**. the hen is stimulated by applying pressure on the lower part of the back with the hand/fingertips. Some hens will respond better to a firm hard stroking motion on the back of the neck from about halfway up the neck down to the back. If the hen lowers her neck slightly into an S-type curve this is an indication of a favorable response. To start with, it may be necessary to hold the wing firmly to slow her down if she tries to get away, until the stimulation makes her stand still. If she does not respond within about 5 minutes, stop and try again later. The most responsive times of the day seemed to be early morning and late evening (this is also the time of day that many emus breed), but some hens are responsive at any time.

The next sign of a positive response from the hen is the raising of the tail feathers. Following this, firm prodding on the tail end with the fingertips and a gentle downward pressure on the back will cause the hen to sit down. Continue to

Plates 12.1 - 12.5 - Stimulation of emus in preparation for artificial insemination. (Photo: J. Groves)

12.1 - Hen raises tail feathers in response to stimulation.

12.2 - Hen sits down while stimulation is continued.

12.3 - "Prodding" around tail area of hen.

12.4 - In this instance the male became interested and was also stimulated.

12.5 - Successful mating. This time artificial insemination was not necessary.

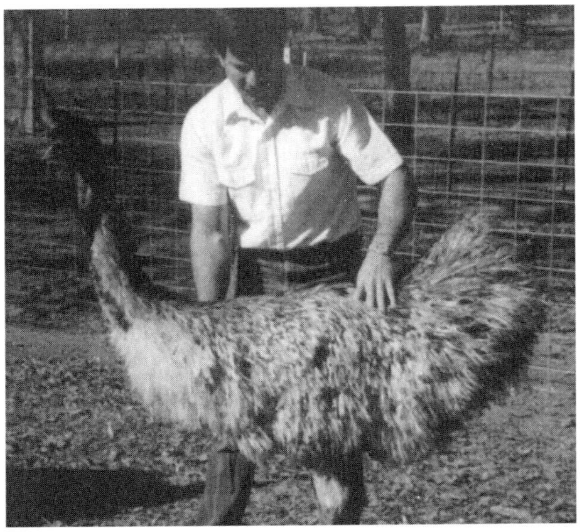

12.1

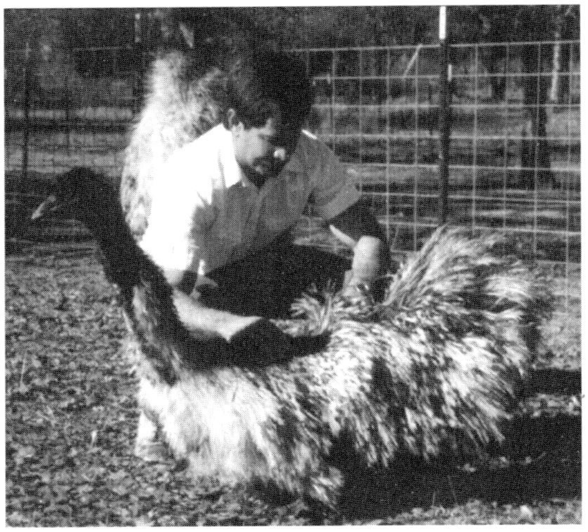

12.2

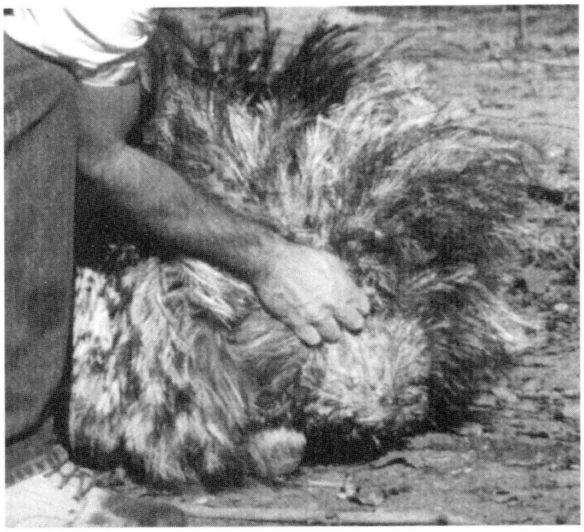

12.3

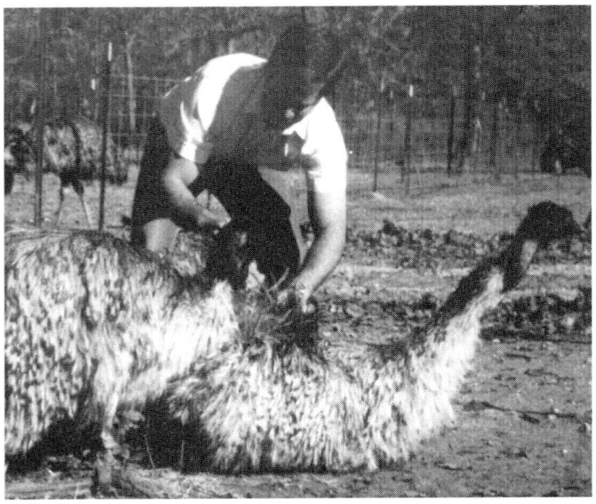

12.4

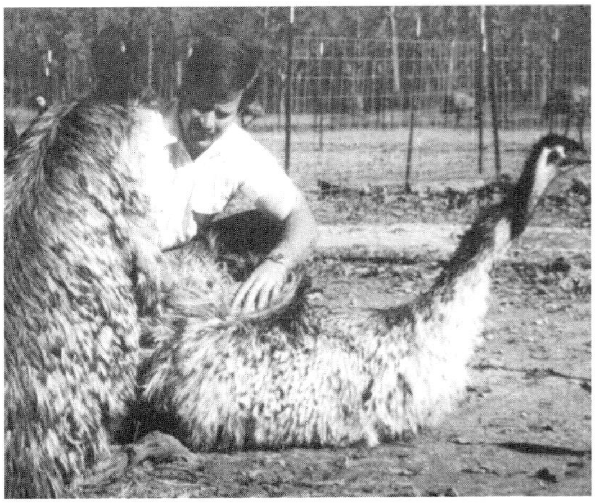

12.5

stroke the back and even pinch the back of the neck with your free hand (simulating the pecking action of the male) until the hen raises her tail in the sitting position. By pushing directly on the cloaca with the palm of the hand, the hen will generally evert the oviduct. This puts it in the correct position for you to insert the syringe full of semen gently about 2 - 3 inches in while holding the everted oviduct with thumb and forefinger, and squeeze the semen into the bird. Gently release, and remove the syringe when she pulls the oviduct back. The insemination is now complete. Back away quietly to allow the hen to get up in her own time.

Note that some hens will evert the oviduct just with the back stimulation. It must protrude about $^1\!/_2$- 1 inch for insemination to be accomplished successfully.

12.5 COMMON REASONS FOR UNSUCCESSFUL INSEMINATION

Since it is still in a very recent stage of research, the artificial insemination of emus is not without problems. The more commonly known reasons for failure or poor rates of success are:

1. Inexperience with the process of insemination (should improve with practice).

2. Wild or nervous birds - need to be tamed down first.

3. Unsuitable semen, e.g. contaminated with feces. Proper handling, patience and practice will help.

4. Improper insemination of hen, or problem with hen which makes her less easily impregnable. If the oviduct is not fully exposed it may not be open to accept the semen. Instead, the semen goes into the cloaca and fertilization does not take place. Often very fat hens have trouble exposing their oviduct fully.

12.6 INSEMINATION INTERVALS

Since we do not yet know how long the sperm can remain alive and active inside the hen, it is recommended to start by inseminating the laying hen 3 days in a row so that the bird is inseminated before and after laying an egg. Then inseminate once every 5 to 7 days. If any infertility shows up later (when the eggs become due to hatch), inseminate more frequently. Generally one should be able to go longer between inseminations and still have good fertility. All birds are individuals however, so conditions will vary. In time, once the emu has been selectively bred for better conformity within the species like any other commercial livestock, results with artificial insemination will also become more similar between hens.

It is always a good idea to solicit the advice and assistance of an interested veterinarian when first starting out.

CHAPTER 13

Problems in the Laying Hen

13.1 INTRODUCTION

In most species of birds, the nutritional needs of the female before and during egg production are quite different from the needs of the male. While both birds need good, balanced diets with enough vitamins and minerals to meet the additional needs of sperm production and yolk/albumen production, the hen has an additional large need for CALCIUM for use in encasing each egg she lays with a strong, hard shell. Eggshell consists of calcium carbonate, to which pigment is added in the oviduct depending on the species or variety of bird. Limestone is also made up of calcium carbonate, as is oystershell.

Since only the female needs the extra calcium, it makes sense to keep the diet balanced to meet the needs of both birds but without the excess calcium, and then to allow the female to satisfy her calcium needs by providing an extra source of calcium free-choice. The limestone or oystershell or crushed eggshell should therefore be placed in a separate location from the feed in the pen, and hopefully the female will consume what she needs. It is important to keep grit/small stones/pebbles in the pen also, as always, because otherwise the male may start to consume the calcium supplement in order to try and satisfy his need for grit. This would not be good for him. The female might also end up over-consuming the supplement, for the same reason.

In poultry, the hen is able to utilize large amounts of calcium in the diet by storing it in the medullary bone. Her weight before the laying season may increase by as much as 20% due to this storage. Possibly emu females are often heavier than the males for the same reason.

Whereas the normal calcium-to-phosphorus ratio in the feed of most animals should be about 1:1 to 2:1, studies done in poultry indicate that a hen can successfully assimilate calcium in as much as a 6:1 ratio - a level at which many other non-egg-laying animals would start to have problems with both calcium and phosphorus absorption, since the two are so inter-related.

The only situation in which it would be justifiable to add calcium to the feed in this higher ratio rather than to just add it as a supplement on the side, would be under artificial insemination conditions, since in such cases there would be no male to worry about.

The vitamin which is most important in the proper assimilation of both calcium and phosphorus by a bird's body, is Vitamin D3. It stands to reason that the laying hen would have a fairly high Vitamin D3 requirement, possibly higher than the male, since she is metabolizing so much calcium. Since a lot of any animal's vitamin D needs are met by sunlight, and since emus lay during winter when there are less hours of sunlight and the weather is often cloudy or rainy (blocking the sun's beneficial rays), some laying problems are no doubt associated with insufficient Vitamin D3. If enough does not seem to be provided by the diet, a supplement (usually given in the form of Vitamins A and D) should be provided, at least during extended periods of sunless weather.

13.2 SOFT-SHELLED EGGS

Many emu hens lay one or two soft-shelled eggs during the course of the breeding season. There is no cause for alarm if the majority of her eggs are normal, lose weight within reasonable levels and hatch out healthy chicks. A large number of soft-shelled or very thin-shelled eggs, however, can indicate that she is not getting (or absorbing) enough calcium from her diet. If there is a plentiful supply of calcium in the form of limestone/oystershell, and the diet seems normally balanced otherwise, giving extra Vit. D3 as well over a period of time may help.

It is also possible that there is a problem in the oviduct such as inflammation or infection, in which case the bird can be put on a course of the appropriate antibiotics. Another possibility is a gut problem, which can lead to poor assimilation of nutrients from the diet. If not much of a calcium store was laid down in the medullary bone prior to laying season, the hen is relying mainly on the diet to supply calcium. If she has an intestinal parasite or other problem that is not making her actually ill, but causes her to utilize her food poorly, she should first be wormed and possibly treated with an antibiotic which works well in gut problems, and then be given some yogurt mixed in with her feed. Not only will this ensure the growth of good bacteria in the stomach, but also it is an immediate source of good nutrients including calcium and phosphorus.

In poultry hens on a diet deficient in Vit. D3 or calcium, the hens not only lay eggs with a thinner and thinner shell but may also deplete their own bones in order to continue laying, to such an extent that they develop fragile bones which break easily (a form of osteoporosis). While we have not as yet observed any such drastic signs in emu females, this does not mean it cannot happen. Certainly a weakening of the bones is possible, perhaps not apparent immediately but leading to problems later on, as with humans who develop osteoporosis. Possibly, however, the emu female would stop laying eggs before robbing her bones of calcium to such an extent.

13.3 INFERTILE EGGS

The problem of infertile eggs is actually not usually a female problem: it is a

MALE problem. After all, the female is not infertile: she is producing the eggs. The male is supposed to produce the sperm to fertilize these eggs, and he is not doing his job. The only way that the female can be held responsible for infertile eggs is if she is not allowing the male to breed her. This kind of incompatibility is best solved either by exchanging her male for another one, or by artificially inseminating the female (see **Chapter 12** on Artificial Insemination.)

However, if the birds are seen breeding and the result is still infertile eggs, a semen sample should be collected from the male (as described in **Section 12.2**) and be checked for problems (dead sperm, deformed sperm etc.) Even if they are not seen breeding, a semen sample could be checked just to make sure. After all, they could be breeding when no-one is around.

Many older males begin to have less viable sperm as they age, and this may in fact be a nutritional problem. Most feed companies and even emu farmers have been looking only at the female's nutritional needs for egg production and have put together diets accordingly, while the male's needs - just as important since without him there will be no chicks - have been overlooked. Many people have therefore been feeding their breeders (both male and female) a high-calcium pellet which is in fact geared mainly to the female. For the male, it may actually be detrimental.

Laying diets that contain more than 2½% calcium (most are significantly higher) with a phosphorus level that makes the calcium-phosphorus ratio abnormally high, e.g. 3:1, 4:1 or higher, can have long-term ill effects on the male bird. Eventually, his kidneys will shut down, but before that, sperm production is affected, becoming less and less. A typical scenario is one of a breeder pair that has been together for 3 years. The first year, production was average but fertility good. The second year, on a different "breeder pellet" (with higher calcium) there were more eggs, but fertility poorer. Finally, the third year the female laid very well, but with NO fertility. What went wrong? A semen sample from the male should clarify the picture, (unless the birds simply are no longer breeding) and a change of diet be made back to a more reasonable calcium-phosphorus ratio. Fortunately, sperm production can come back, given a better diet. Hopefully, the problem will be corrected before any lasting damage to the kidneys is done, since they do not have as much regenerative power.

Of course, this is not the only problem that has the potential to cause male infertility, but it is certainly one worth considering. Obesity in one or both of the breeders can also contribute to infertility, not only because of physical changes (e.g. the hen cannot protrude the oviduct sufficiently for proper mating) but because birds sometimes become too lethargic to breed.

13.4 THE EGG-BOUND HEN

Occasionally a hen which has been on a regular laying cycle becomes "egg-bound", i.e. is unable to lay the egg for some reason. It remains stuck in the lower part of the oviduct, usually the uterus, and the bird is seen to sit down and stand up repeatedly as her attempts to lay continue to be futile. She may not eat, appears generally uncomfortable and stands hunched. This is not a very common occurrence among emus, but a few cases have been seen.

Egg-binding in any bird tends to occur more when the weather is cold, no doubt because the bird's metabolism has slowed down and so the muscular movements that bring the egg down the oviduct have also slowed. The egg may also be somewhat larger than usual, which might not be a problem when the weather is warm and the bird in good shape, but can add to the problem under the conditions that promote egg-binding.

When egg-binding is suspected, not only because the egg is overdue but also because the hen appears uncomfortable, the following treatment usually helps:

1. Try to warm up the bird, e.g. by closing her up and hanging a heat lamp in her shelter if the weather is still cold. If a heating pad is available, it may also be used.

2. Using warmed-up K-Y jelly or mineral oil generously grease the bird's cloaca and try to squirt the lubricant as far up into the bird as is possible, in the hope that some will work its way up the oviduct. Be gentle, and gently massage the area also. By inserting a finger into the cloaca, the egg can usually be felt. Lubrication and massage alone may help.

3. Give the bird a calcium injection e.g. calcium gluconate (or have the veterinarian give it.) Egg binding is often associated with low blood calcium, so this generally helps.

4. If necessary, a shot of pitocin can also be administered by the vet. This should help to get the muscles around the oviduct contracting.

Usually, given these treatments, the bird should be able to lay the egg within a day or sooner. Keep her quiet and warm.

If nothing happens, surgical intervention can be done to remove the egg from the oviduct but it should only be tried as an absolute last resort. Also be sure that what you are feeling is in fact an egg, and not the tip of the tailbone or other bone. This mistake has been made before. The skeleton drawing **(Fig. 4.1)** can be helpful in determining where the bones actually are. An X-ray may be helpful prior to surgery, to determine whether a second egg is also present in the oviduct, which could cause complications. Should surgery be necessary, general anesthesia should be used and the 3" to 4" incision be made on the left side, about 3" up from the bird's ventral mid-line, having first located the egg by palpating from side and/or through cloaca. Carefully remove egg, sew up oviduct with absorbable sutures and then close the incision. The very elastic nature of the oviduct should ensure that normal egg-laying will still be possible in future, in spite of the growth of some scar tissue.

It is possible for a veterinarian to remove an egg that is stuck by crushing it in the oviduct and attempting to aspirate most of its contents. Given the hard shell of an emu egg, not only is this a difficult procedure but it is also fraught with danger for the bird, as shell pieces could puncture the oviduct and cause even greater problems.

13.5 EGG YOLK PERITONITIS

Egg yolk peritonitis, although sometimes loosely called "egg-binding" as well, is a very different condition from egg-binding and seems to occur most frequently in hens which are too fat. Instead of dropping into the funnel of the oviduct, the ovum (egg yolk) misses and falls into the stomach cavity, where it is treated as a foreign body and causes peritonitis. The body will attempt to encapsulate the egg so that when such eggs are removed from the stomach cavity they are encased in white secretions and do not much resemble an egg. They have been mistaken for abscesses on occasion, as they look similar. Unfortunately, once one ovum has dropped into the wrong place, others are likely to follow since often what has happened is that the extra fat on the bird has displaced the funnel of the oviduct or caused its lip to fold over in such a way that it cannot catch the ovum.

If the bird's body successfully encapsulates each of the ova, she may appear to recover after looking ill for a while, although of course she will not lay any more eggs that season. However, any hard knock that she receives could burst one of these eggs in the abdomen and set up a peritonitis too severe to recover from. **Plate 13.1** shows such a bird, which had appeared normal until subjected to the stress of being loaded in a trailer and moved. She had nine encapsulated egg yolks in her stomach cavity.

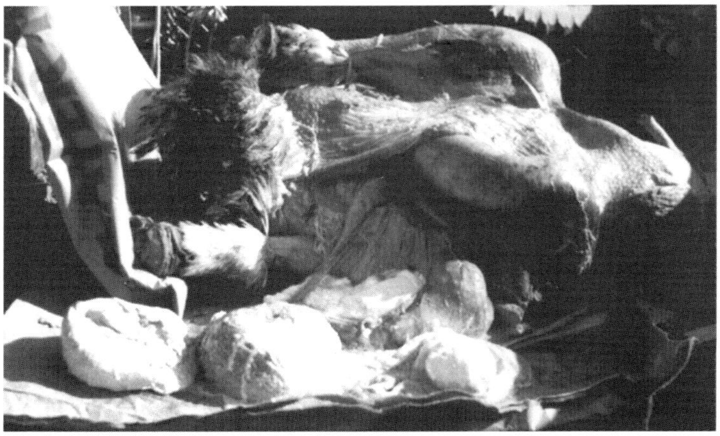

Plate 13.1 - Encapsulated egg yolks in abdomen of female which died from egg yolk peritonitis.

In egg yolk peritonitis, the encapsulated eggs can usually be palpated by gently feeling the bird's abdomen and belly, as they will generally settle to the bottom of the stomach cavity. They are of course not the normal egg shape but are felt as independent chunks of matter that can easily be moved around. They should be removed by surgery and the bird be given a course of antibiotics. If the bird recovers from surgery and is given plenty of exercise to slim down (as well as feeding her less) she may recover to lay eggs in the normal way again. There is no recourse other than surgery for egg yolk peritonitis.

13.6 PROLAPSED OVIDUCT/CLOACA

Very occasionally, for reasons unknown, a female bird may have the latter part of her oviduct prolapse, via the cloaca. **Plate 13.2** of color section shows an example of this. **Treatment**: Catch the bird, strap the legs together and lay it on the ground as outlined in **Section 3.2**. With an assistant holding the bird still, wash the prolapsed oviduct with Betadine solution and gently push it back into the cloaca. Do not try to invert it while it is outside the bird. Hold it in place for a few minutes and proceed to put a strong purse-string stitch around the anus using silk thread. Be sure to leave about 3/4" or the thickness of a man's index finger open for the bird to defecate through. Treat the bird with an antibiotic for a full course. Remove the stitch at about 8-10 days. Watch the bird closely for a week afterwards to be sure normal bowel movements occur. The bird should resume normal laying in a few months (by the next season).

CHAPTER 14

Treatment of Diseases and Injuries

While good management techniques and good nutrition can do a lot to reduce the incidence of disease and injury to livestock, it is inevitable that these problems will sometimes occur. This is as true in emu farming as in the farming of any other type of animal. For this reason it is important to have a good relationship with a veterinarian who is willing to work with and educate himself about emus. This chapter is intended as an aid to both emu farmers and veterinarians as it describes health problems seen to date in emus and methods that have been used in their treatment.

It should be noted that because the field of emu medicine is so new, there are no medications which have been specifically registered as safe for use in emus. For this reason, some veterinarians will require a written waiver by the emu farmer before dispensing certain medications. This is a reasonable request which should cause no problems to either party. Finally, it is likely that when the emu becomes classified as a food animal, many drug restrictions will begin to apply to it as to other livestock raised for slaughter, to ensure the absence of drug residues in the meat.

14.1 RECOGNIZING SIGNS OF ILLNESS

Other than the obviously visible symptoms of injury seen in emus with fractures, cuts, lacerations and severe bites/stings, the general signs of illness in an emu include:

- standing hunched up or lying down on its own rather than moving around with the other birds in the group
- not eating (although may stand with other birds at the feed trough)
- loss of vigor - does not struggle in the normal way when held, handled or picked up (chick).
- dull, brittle feathers and stunted growth (signs of a chronic problem, i.e. one that develops over a longer period of time.)

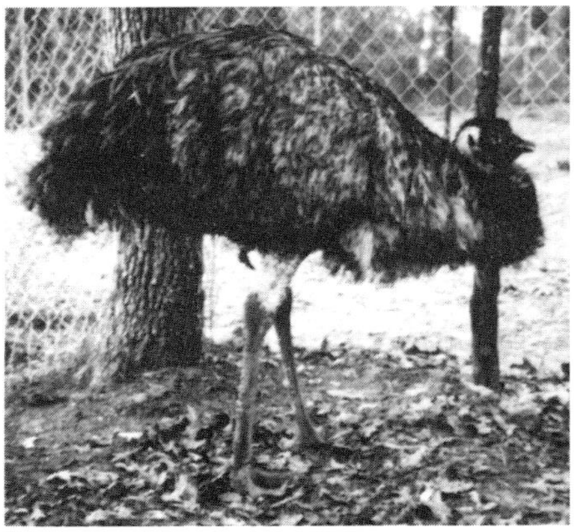

Plate 14.1 - Typical "hunched" position of sick bird.

More specific symptoms which pertain to different problems are outlined in the sections that follow.

14.2 WORKING WITH YOUR VETERINARIAN

Since most veterinarians have had no training in the field of emu medicine, and most emu farmers have tried to educate themselves about their birds in every way they can, the relationship between the emu farmer and his veterinarian should involve pooling their resources, in the best interests of the birds. There are many medical treatments, such as stitching up injured animals, which apply to most animal species and for which the veterinarian is well trained and equipped. He/she also has good resources in the form of many textbooks, informed colleagues and university staff to research possible causes for different illnesses, and make a diagnosis based on an educated opinion.

The emu farmer, in turn, can help by providing his veterinarian with as much relevant emu information as he can; by giving the veterinarian the opportunity to familiarize himself/herself with the birds under normal conditions, as well as providing fresh carcasses of any birds that die for study by autopsy; by restraining the bird properly when the vet wishes to examine it; and by providing accurate clinical histories on birds as needed, by observing them closely on a regular basis and noting any unusual signs.

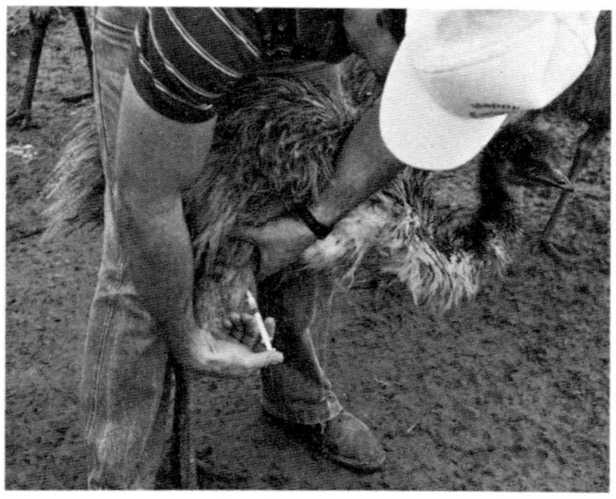

Plate 14.2 - Injecting young bird.

If the veterinarian is going to be called out to see a bird, it is usually better not to medicate it until he/she has seen it, if this is at all possible. Some medications mask the symptoms of disease, and it will be more helpful to the vet in making a diagnosis if the bird can first be seen before any treatment is done.

Drawing Conclusions: The Importance of "Controls"

It is wise not to jump to any conclusions about what must be wrong with a sick bird, because if every angle of the problem is not considered, one could miss something that is quite obvious and give the bird a treatment that will not help at all. Stool samples which the veterinarian can check for intestinal parasites, blood samples and bacterial cultures are all useful tools which should be taken advantage of when a diagnosis is uncertain.

Even when a bird is treated with medication and gets well, one should still be open to the possibility that the bird might have improved even without the medication, and therefore the fact that he appeared to respond to it does not mean that he did. One cannot assume that a medication actually helped unless there is another bird, suffering from the same problem, that can be used as a "control" in that it is not medicated. If the medicated bird recovers and the unmedicated one does not, then one is reasonably safe to assume that the diagnosis of the problem was correct and that the medication helped the bird. Cases of birds being treated without the use of controls have led to many erroneous conclusions as to causes and treatments of different problems - there have been many cases where birds have improved **in spite of** the "treatment" rather than **because** of it. An objective outlook is therefore essential, as well as an honest appraisal of how much one actually does know.

14.3 INJURY

(a) Lacerations to the Body

When adult birds fight and are not separated, some serious injuries can result especially if they are in a small pen with nowhere to hide. The aggressor often kicks deep gashes into the back and sides of her or his mate. There is often bruising and featherless patches, and by the time the wounded bird is discovered and separated, he is usually panting heavily and obviously stressed. Some wounds may be due to running into the fence in an attempt to escape.

Fortunately, even the worst-looking wounds of this nature often heal quite rapidly, especially in locations where the fat-layer is quite thick underneath. Generally, stitching is not required, but the application of antiseptic spray or powder is recommended. It is usually best to leave the wounds open, once treated, so that they can dry and heal. New black feather growth will start to occur in the bare patches within a week or two. A course of broad-spectrum antibiotics is a good idea, e.g. penicillin or tetracycline, in order to curb any infection of the wounds. To be effective, any antibiotic must be given for a full course (minimum is usually 3 -5 days) even if the bird appears to have recovered before this.

(b) Lacerations to the Neck

Neck injuries are more serious, and can occur through fighting, attack by dogs, entanglement in wire or can be self-inflicted when the bird is struggling to get out of a handler's grasp and rips his neck with his own foot (see **Section 3.4**). Sometimes the bird's esophagus is torn, sometimes the trachea, and occasionally both.

The bird is usually given a general anesthetic (e.g. Rompun/Ketamine or Telazol) and after the area is cleaned with Betadine solution, the esophagus or trachea is stitched using absorbable sutures and the neck skin closed. The veterinarian should be made aware of the natural opening in the trachea (used for vocalization) so that he does not stitch it closed also, which would probably make the bird unable to boom or grunt.

Provided the damage is not too extensive, many emus make a good recovery. A course of antibiotics after the operation is a normal precaution against infection,

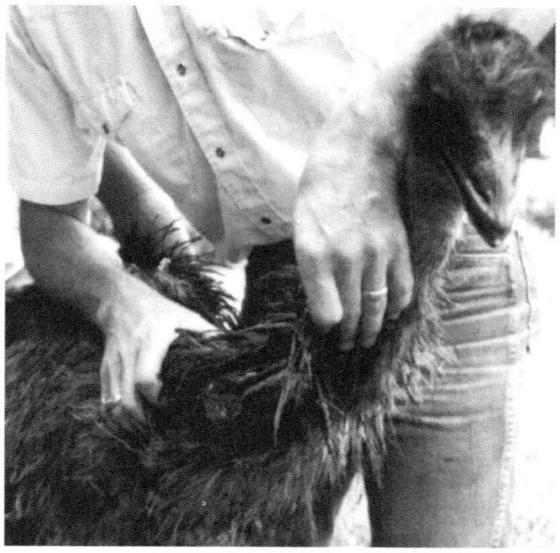

Plate 14.3 (a) - Bird with torn neck and esophagus due to injury.

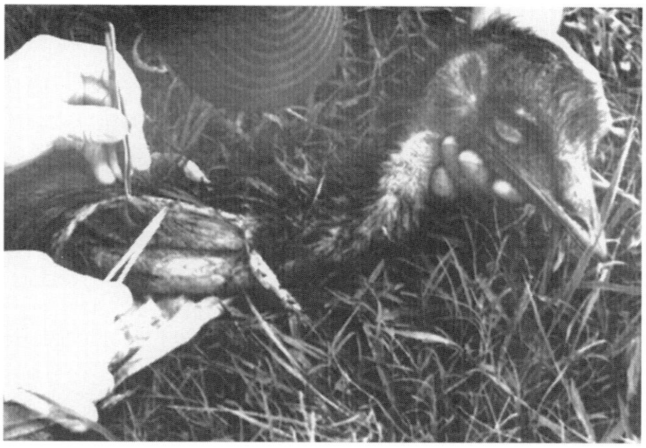

Plate 14.3 (b) - Stitching torn esophagus while bird is under anesthesia.

and the bird should be closely observed to make sure he is drinking water. He may not eat for a few days but this is not usually a problem. Adding cracked corn to the diet may help the bird resume eating sooner, by providing additional visual stimulation.

(c) Deep Puncture Wounds

Any bird that has run into a fence or otherwise injured himself should also be checked for deep puncture wounds. These are the more dangerous because they are not so readily apparent amongst the bird's thick feathers. Since deep wounds usually do not bleed much (thereby flushing out many bacteria), infection can develop more easily and can lead to a condition known as "gas-gangrene", where the tissues become swollen, soft and spongy around the site of the infection. By the time this sets in, the condition is very serious, and the bird should immediately be started on a course of penicillin (injectable, for faster effect). Also treat the wound by opening and flushing it.

Because it is easy to overlook a puncture wound, it is a good precaution to put any bird that has been injured on a course of antibiotics.

(d) Leg Bands Outgrown

It is important to keep a periodic check on leg bands used on young, growing birds. As a chick goes through a growth spurt, the leg thickens and the result can be a leg band that is so tight that it starts cutting into the flesh. The bird then begins to limp and the leg may swell up on either side of the band.

The bird should be restrained, the leg band carefully cut off and any broken skin swabbed with iodine (Betadine) solution. The swelling, limping and indentation in the flesh usually start to improve within just a few days.

(e) Injuries due to Cannibalism

Any chick in a group which has a bare patch of skin, a small sore or some other area of visual contrast on its head or body, is in danger of being "cannibalized" by the other chicks particularly when they are confined in a smaller area.The chicks are very attracted to the contrasting spot and tend to peck at it as much as they can. This can make a tiny scratch into a large ugly wound, which of course is even more attractive for the chicks to peck at.

Prevention of cannibalism includes such measures as keeping smaller groups of chicks together, especially when they have to be confined for any length of time e.g. during bad weather; making sure all chicks in a group are about the same size; keeping lights dim in an area of confinement; and providing shiny or brightly colored alternative "targets" for chicks to peck at. The target can be a brightly colored ball, a child's toy suspended above the pen (adding the stimulus of movement to that of color, contrast and brightness) or anything which is visually stimulating but that the birds are unable to swallow. Of course, the best prevention of all is to allow chicks a good-sized outside run with plenty of natural vegetation, rocks and stones to keep them busy pecking at other things all day. Feeding should also be done on a regular schedule so that chicks do not start pecking at each other because they are hungry and expecting food. A dietary deficiency could also be a cause of cannibalism, as the birds try to find a source of the nutrient(s) which they lack.

Treatment of a bird that has been "cannibalized" includes making the sore less visible as well as disinfecting it. Betadine solution is useful in both respects, since it tends to make the area brown. The chick can also be separated or even placed in a group of slightly smaller chicks, which will not tend to peck on the larger one. The most often "cannibalized" areas are the beak, head and back. Some emu farmers have used "superglue" to attach feathers to bare skin patches around wounds. This also helps make these areas less visible.

In the worst case seen, the chick was pecked raw on the head as far as the skull and on the side of the face right down to the bone and eyelids. The wounds were putrid, but the chick was very energetic. It was given a course of antibiotics (injectable), separated from the other chicks and swabbed twice daily with a mixture of DMSO (dimethyl sulfoxide) and furazone. Amazingly, it made a complete recovery, did not lose the eye but grew a cone-shaped area of skin around the affected eye in place of eyelids, and grew up to be a good male breeder. Since his disfigurement was not hereditary but caused by injury, there was no reason not to use him in the breeding program.

(f) Internal Injuries/Bruising

A bird with internal injuries through experiencing a severe blow, e.g. by running into something (fence-post, other solid obstruction) will usually appear listless and unwell, and may not want to eat. If a lot of blood has been lost as a result of internal bleeding, it will be anemic as well.

Other than general support therapy (see **Section 14.8(f)**) to help combat stress, the bird can be injected with Vitamin B12 to help build up blood again. An iron supplement may also be given. An anti-inflammatory injection (e.g. Banamine) usually helps the bird feel better and reduces any swelling, and a course of antibiotics is also a good idea. Each case should of course be assessed individually, and the assistance of a good veterinarian can be very helpful.

Injury to **kidneys** may occur from a bird falling very hard on its back; from the inappropriate use of certain drugs such as Amikacin or Gentamicin (antibiotics) when the bird was very dehydrated; or from infective agents. An inflamed (swollen) kidney may result in limping and difficulty in walking because of the extreme pain.

If kidney damage is so severe that no (white) urates are being passed along with stool, and the bird appears extremely sick, chances for recovery are not good. Once kidneys shut down completely, the body can no longer function.

14.4 TREATMENT OF FRACTURES AND LEG DEFORMITIES

While most "splayed leg" conditions in emu chicks appear to be related to nutritional deficiencies, others can be due to injury, e.g. dislocation or injury to ligaments in hip from slipping on a slick surface. Attempts have been made to surgically correct this problem. However, the pinning and plating of bones in most ratites, including emus, in order to correct deformities or attempt to set broken legs, has usually met with only a limited degree of success. This is partly because the spongy nature of the inside (medulla) of the bone does not lend itself readily to this method, and partly because the nature of the bird itself does not allow for long periods of quiet rest or for very careful use of the injured part. Rather, the bird will struggle mightily to rid himself of any encumbrance and attempt to run, no matter how much pain this may cause him. Pins tend to pull out of bones easily because of these factors. Placing a bird in a sling to allow him time to heal is also usually an unsatisfactory method, since it takes a lot of time and labor to maintain a bird in this situation and causes a lot of stress to him too. Muscles may also atrophy since the bird is not walking. Breathing is sometimes difficult for a bird in a sling because of the pressure on the chest and sides.

In the case of leg deformities that are not too severe and that have been caused by nutritional deficiencies, methods of correction that are less drastic and invasive such as bone-scraping (to increase bone growth in desired places) may be a better alternative than breaking, rotating and pinning the bone. Aftercare in the latter case is extremely difficult and time-consuming, whereas in the former case the bird is allowed to walk right away.

Braces, harnesses and splints to try to correct twisted-leg problems usually are not successful since they seem to interfere with the bird's center of gravity more than anything else and do not correct the underlying problem. However, a **small** problem such as a folded-over foot in a young chick can be treated by taping an L-shaped splint under the foot and up the back of the leg.

The best way to deal with leg deformities is to try to prevent them by correct nutrition. Most severe cases have to be euthanatized eventually. As for fractures, unless they are of a nature where the leg can be strapped with an elastic bandage for support and the bird can still get around in this way, it makes better farming sense to euthanatize the bird.

14.5 PROBLEMS INVOLVING THE DIGESTIVE TRACT

(a) Impaction /Ingestion of foreign objects

Impaction is a problem that does not occur as commonly in emus as in ostriches or rheas. This may be due to the different structure of the gut and faster time of food passage in emus. Impaction occurs when there is a complete or partial blockage in the gut (usually the gizzard) due to the presence of some inappropriate material which the bird has ingested. In the emu, the most common material to cause impaction is long fibrous matter such as long grass stems, synthetic fibers picked from carpeting, and string. It is not usual for the emu to impact on sand or dirt; these tend to pass through the gut fairly easily.

Three situations that predispose a bird to impaction are:

1. Irregular feeding routine or omitted feedings, together with

2. The presence of some fibrous material (carpeting, long dry grass, thin sticks, etc.)

3. Lack of small stones or gravel to use as "teeth" in the gizzard (i.e. to help grind up food).

The offending material cannot be moved on through the gut and causes a "traffic jam" of sorts. Long grass fibers may be laying longitudinally in the gut or gizzard and cannot be moved on; string often balls up into a clump.

Treatment by tubing with water and a fiber laxative (e.g. Metamucil) or mineral oil is usually successful. The fiber laxative will cause long fibrous material to bind together better, and will also help its progress through the gut.

Mineral oil helps move impacted material by generously lubricating it. Two to four treatments may be needed at intervals of 6 to 12 hours in order to successfully clear the impaction. When mineral oil is used, the stool will be shiny and oily as the oil passes through. Mineral oil does not stimulate a cough reflex and is easily aspirated, so make sure the tube is well down the esophagus and past the opening of the trachea. (See **Section 14.10**, Tube Feeding).

A very severe impaction which does not respond to tubing can be treated with surgery (cutting gizzard open and removing the offending material). This should be done by a qualified veterinarian.

Impacted birds are generally listless, stand hunched up, do not eat or drink much if at all, and pass little or no stool. The gizzard often feels hard and **remains** hard, unlike birds who have just eaten whose gizzards feel full and hard at first, but become soft in a few hours as the food is digested.

Ingestion of foreign material can sometimes cause impaction, as described. In other cases it passes through with no harm to the bird. Birds have been known to eat and pass pieces of glass with no internal damage. However, if a sharp object punctures the gut, this is a serious problem. A very small puncture may heal on its own; a larger hole, however, generally causes peritonitis as stomach contents leak out into the abdominal cavity. Since often, not even an X-ray will reveal where the hole in the gut is so that a surgical repair can be attempted, chances of recovery for a bird with a punctured gut are not good. A bird in this condition will grow more and more emaciated, even though he may eat and drink. His feathers become dull and brittle, he may walk with difficulty or stagger around from weakness and pain, and treatment with antibiotics usually does not help. The bird eventually dies, and should then be autopsied to confirm the diagnosis and to rule out other actual diseases that cause similar chronic symptoms.

(b) Intestinal Parasites

Although emus in general (in the U.S.) do not often seem to have health problems with intestinal worms/other parasites, a few cases have been recorded. Most have involved protozoan parasites rather than worms, and have mainly occurred where birds were being raised under unsanitary conditions or in old poultry facilities which had not been properly cleaned and disinfected. **Coccidiosis**, which is characterized by blood in the stool in its more advanced stages, can be treated with amprolium.

Histomoniasis (also known as "blackhead" infection in turkeys, where it invades the ceca and the liver) has been successfully treated with dimetridazole (Emtryl).

Because stool samples did not often reveal problems with worm infestation in emus, it was not thought necessary at first to worm these birds. However, after the discovery of a small roundworm which invades the spinal cord and brain of (young) emus, as described in **Section 14.6**, most emu farmers are now worming their birds on a regular basis.

(c) Bacterial and Viral Infections Involving The Gut

In addition to the gastro-intestinal problems already described, gut problems in emus may also be BACTERIAL or VIRAL in origin. Chicks around the age of 3 weeks tend to be the most susceptible to acute bacterial or viral infections, since it is around this time that the contents of the yolk sac - including maternal antibodies - have been completely absorbed. The chick's own immune system is usually not yet well developed at this stage. Of course, the better the bird's state of nutrition and general health, the better chance it has of fighting off any infection. Cleanliness and insect control are also especially important during this period, since many insects are carriers of disease.

Any change in stool may be indicative of a gut problem. For this reason routine observation of the stool is important (see **Section 14.9**).

If **bacterial** enteritis is suspected, it should be treated with an appropriate antibiotic as soon as possible. Injectable Di-Trim (trimethoprim/sulfadiazine) or the sulfa drugs are often used with success. Old, stagnant water can become contaminated with bacteria and cause such problems. If the problem is left untreated for too long, the continual straining can cause PROLAPSE of the end portion of the intestine, as described further on in the text.

Viruses can also cause an acute gastro-enteritis. The most dangerous viral illness seen in emus to date in the U.S. is **Eastern equine encephalomyelitis** (abbreviated EEE) which has been known to occur in many other species of birds as well, in addition to horses and even man. Instead of showing symptoms typical to diseases of the brain/spinal cord such as derangement and listless or abnormal behavior, the disease in emus is very sudden and acute. Bloody diarrhea is followed by extreme debilitation and then death, sometimes within the day. Intensive support therapy is about the only treatment, and will not always work. In the few birds that were able to make a complete recovery from EEE, the very intensive support therapy included oral doses of Pepto-Bismol to help coat the severly traumatized intestinal tract as well as tube-feeding (vitamins/electrolytes/nutrients); antibiotics to combat any secondary infections; Banamine for pain; and intravenous fluids (Lactated Ringer's Solution/Dextrose solution) by means of a jugular catheter. The jugular catheter was inserted at the first onset of bloody diarrhea, in a similar manner to drawing blood (see **Section 14.11**). Most birds affected were over a year old. Vaccination of emus with the killed vaccine used for horses will hopefully prevent the disease, although research is still underway to find out how effective the vaccine is in emus, and for how long. The disease is seasonal, being carried by biting insects (certain species of mosquitoes), which also means that it will occur more in swampy, low-lying areas with large populations of carrier mosquitoes, especially after a mild winter/wet spring.

The likelihood of there being EEE cases during winter is reduced, since there are fewer mosquitoes around at that time. The disease was first diagnosed in emus by Louisiana State University, School of Veterinary Medicine (Baton Rouge, Louisiana) where research on its prevention in emus by the use of vaccine is continuing. The vaccine being used also protects against two other types of equine encephalomyelitis, Western and Venezuelan (abbreviated WEE and VEE). While not as serious as EEE, cases of WEE have now also been positively diagnosed in emus. Symptoms are mainly neurological, e.g. staggering, weakness and disorientation.

(d) Vent Prolapse

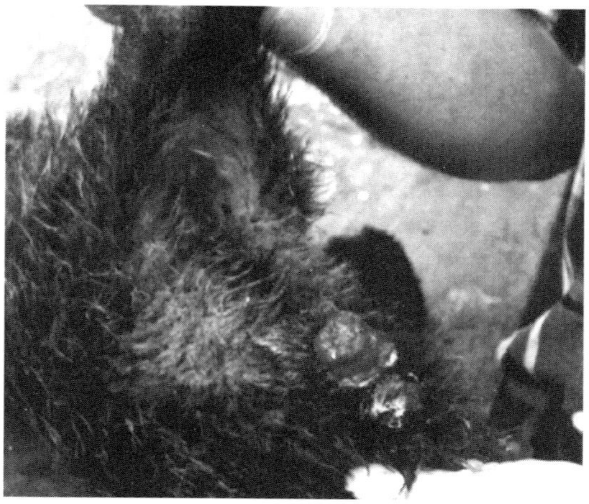

Plate 14.4 - Vent prolapse in 2-to 3-month-old chick (before treatment).

In some severe gastro-intestinal infections, emu chicks may do so much straining in the passing of stool that there is a prolapse, i.e. the final part of the intestine (cloaca) everts and hangs out of the vent, as shown in **Plate 14.4**. This can also happen in extreme constipation. Of course, the underlying problem (whether diarrhea or constipation) must be found and treated, e.g. with Metamucil or mineral oil and antibiotics, and the prolapsed portion must be swabbed clean with Betadine and pushed back in through the vent. If it prolapses again, a purse-string stitch may be needed for a few days (as in the case of prolapsed oviduct, **Section 13.6**). The bird should be carefully watched to make sure he is able to pass stool in spite of the stitch. If he seems to be straining and unable to pass stool, the stitch can be taken out or loosened, then redone after stool has been passed. The stitch is removed as soon as it seems that the cloaca will stay in place. This problem may take some careful nursing, but can generally be corrected.

14.6 UPPER RESPIRATORY AND CENTRAL NERVOUS SYSTEM INFECTIONS

A variety of upper respiratory infections have been seen in emus, notably in groups of emu chicks under 6 months old. It is likely that many such infections are viral, although bacterial sources have also been cultured. Emus may exhibit a variety of the following symptoms:

- Frothy or gummed-up eyes (conjunctivitis)
- "Runny nose" or thick mucus in nostrils (rhinitis, sinusitis)
- Wheezing, labored breathing, inability to chirp (worst cases)— laryngitis, possible air sacculitis
- Phlegm in throat
- Red, inflamed trachea, notably around its opening (tracheitis, possible bronchitis)
- Ataxia (staggering) in conjunction with one or more of these symptoms (possibly due to middle ear infection, meningitis or hypoglycemia).
- Head-pushing (against fence), extreme docility and other abnormal behavior indicating brain is also affected (encephalitis, meningitis)

Treatment is as follows:

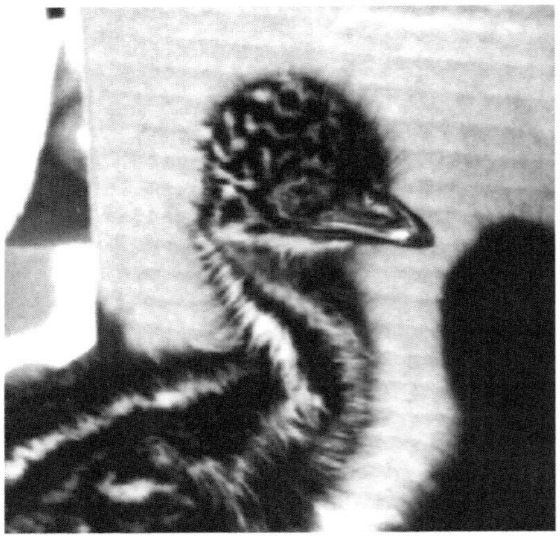

Plate 14.5 - Crusty, gummed-up eye (infected) in small chick.

- Put all birds in group on a course of antibiotics (broad-spectrum, such as Terramycin in drinking water, or Amoxicillin injected sub-cutaneously). Most infections among chicks that start with congestion in the nose or eyes spread quickly to every chick in the group. Therefore, even if all chicks are not yet showing symptoms, it is better to treat them all together. Even if the cause is viral and not bacterial, infection by a virus leaves the bird weakened and wide open to secondary infection by bacteria, so antibiotics are a good precaution.

- Clean affected eyes and nostrils daily with warm saline solution. (A spoonful of table salt dissolved in warm water works fine.) Remove any thick scabs or crustiness to expose the pink flesh underneath, since bacteria can hide under scabs. If nostrils seem blocked, add a little food coloring to the saline solution, squirt this solution into each nostril with a thin syringe (without the needle) and open the beak to see if the food coloring can be observed in the upper palate. It should drain through the slits which connect nostrils with mouth. Once the food coloring is seen, this means the passages are open and medication will be effective. Treat both eyes and nostrils with a few drops of Chloramphenicol or Gentamicin eye drops. This treatment can be repeated twice daily if necessary. Eye ointment such as Terramycin or Chloramphenicol ointment can be used to rub around eyes and soften scabs. A persistent **fungal** infection around eyes can be treated with Nystatin liquid, being careful not to get any in eyes as it will sting.

- Wash all the chicks' backs daily with a mixture of chlorine bleach and warm water. This is to prevent the birds from re-infecting themselves, as their tendency is to rub their eyes and beaks on their backs. The bleach solution should help kill any bacteria deposited on the feathers.

- Support therapy (see **Section 14.8(f)**) may be needed in some of the more severe cases. Acute infections may deplete birds severely, and if there are any signs of weakness such as staggering, feet folding over when the bird walks, or complete lack of interest in food and water, the bird should be tube-fed with a glucose/electrolyte solution, to which some crushed feed or high-protein baby cereal can be added as needed.

- Strict attention to hygiene is important, such as changing bedding in birds' shelter daily and making sure (if hay is used) that the hay is fresh and clean, not moldy or damp. Floors and walls may be cleaned fairly frequently with a safe disinfectant (phenolic compounds are usually good for this) and feeders/waterers cleaned with chlorine bleach solution.

- Insect control, by fogging or placing fans on birds at night or applying a safe insect repellent to their heads and necks, is very important. Biting/bloodsucking insects probably play a large part in the spreading of these upper respiratory diseases, since the incidence is the greatest when the insect problem is at its worst.

Note that there are some Mycoplasma infections which will cause inflammation (swelling, heat) of the joints as well as sinusitis, conjunctivitis and other upper respiratory symptoms. If such signs are seen, treatment with Tylosin (antibiotic) is usually effective. It is available both as a powder which can be dissolved in the drinking water and as the injectable Tylan-200.

Note also that infectious diseases, just like vitamin deficiencies, often do not occur alone. Symptoms of several diseases may be seen, because there are several types of infective organisms involved. A classic case is the combination of upper respiratory symptoms with neurological symptoms (showing brain is affected), e.g.

- Ataxia (also a symptom of low blood sugar levels, of specific nutritional deficiencies such as copper or Vitamin A, and of toxicities)
- head-pushing
- abnormally docile or aggressive behavior
- extreme weakness, disorientation
- temporary blindness
- convulsions (again, this can be a symptom of many other problems too).
- lack of co-ordination, e.g. stumbling, or feet crossing over when walking

All these symptoms have been seen in emus during an especially wet year when insects of every form abounded. Fortunately, with appropriate treatment and support therapy, all birds recovered. Pneumonia is not often seen in emus, although if upper respiratory infections were left untreated, it might easily develop.

There is one recently discovered disease affecting the brain and spinal cord from which birds do **not** easily recover. In addition to the general neurological symptons listed above, this disease also causes a twisted neck and/or back. The problem has mainly been seen in young birds (under a year old) and will make the birds very sick and weak - unlike young birds which get a crooked neck while remaining healthy, whose problem is probably nutritional (**Section 6.6**). This disease is not due to a bacteria or virus, but due to a roundworm (nematode) whose larvae invade the spinal cord and brain of the emu, usually causing death. The emus affected are believed to have become "incidental hosts" to this worm, which is found in some local bird populations and is carried by certain types of biting insects. For this reason, swampy areas with large populations of biting/bloodsucking insects are the highest-risk areas for this disease, as they are for EEE which is also an insect-borne disease (see **Section 14.5(c)**.)

Regular treatment with Ivermectin, which can be injected subcutaneously or given orally, will hopefully help in preventing this problem. In high-risk areas, many emu farmers are worming their birds as often as every 3 weeks. Studies to determine the effectiveness and frequency of worming necessary are still underway. For more detailed information, refer to Blue-McLendon, Alice, et al. 1991. Veterinary Quarterly Review, Texas Veterinary Extension Service.

14.7 BITES AND STINGS

Apart from causing irritation and stress, certain insect bites/stings can be harmful to emus as they can to any other animals, because of the damage done to the tissue itself - especially around head, neck and eyes - and because of the release of toxins into the system.

Severe stinging in and around the eyes is treated like an eye infection (see **Section 14.6**). If the bird seems to be in a lot of pain, Atropine drops can also be instilled, but only late in the evening as it causes pupil dilation and thus could cause damage to eyes in harsh sunlight. Ulcerations around eyes due to stings can be treated with Gentamicin eye ointment, which may be periodically mixed with DMSO (dimethyl sulfoxide) for increased penetration. The use of DMSO is a controversial subject as it is a potent and very penetrating chemical (should be applied using latex gloves), but in cases we have treated, good healing has taken place.

A steroid such Dexamethasone or other anti-inflammatory drug such as Banamine is useful in cases of severe swelling associated with insect stings. Antibiotics and general support therapy should also be used. An injectable or oral antihistamine (e.g. Benadryl) is also a good idea.

External treatment of stings with anti-inflammatory and/or antibiotic ointments can also be helpful. The skin in these areas may eventually slough off and be replaced by new skin. When severe stinging by wasps in particular has taken place, it may be two to three months before the birds look good again. However, with the appropriate treatment there is usually a complete recovery even in the worst cases.

Although emus rarely seem to become infested with external bloodsucking parasites such as ticks/fleas/lice, they can safely be treated with malathion/Sevin dust if such infestations were to occur. Sucking lice can also be controlled by twice-yearly worming with Ivermectin.

14.8 STRESS

"Stress" is defined in the dictionary as "a physical, chemical or emotional factor that causes bodily or mental tension and may be a factor in causing disease." One of the many challenges of farming any animal is to provide an environment that is as stress-free as possible, since any animal that is under continual stress will not grow as well or produce as well as one that is unstressed and content.

Obviously it is not possible to keep all emus calm and quiet all of the time. Birds have to be moved, fed, watered, eggs collected etc. They may also take fright at strange noises or sounds. Chasing or even fighting may occur, especially amongst groups of young birds approaching sexual maturity.

Short periods of stress like these usually do no harm; in fact, it is even possible that some of this behavior might stimulate the mating urge. However, any prolonged periods of stress can be harmful and need to be managed in the appropriate way.

(a) Signs of Stress

Emus usually show stress in one of two ways:

1. Excessive, nervous pacing or running along the fence, sometimes pushing hard against it or even running into it. Young chicks may also give loud, piercing "distress calls", whistling in two to three short bursts at a time.

2. Depression - standing or sitting around, not eating, drinking or participating in any of the activity seen in other birds around it. This is often not recognized immediately since the bird is calling no attention to himself, but is a sign of stress or illness which a farmer needs to be very aware of.

(b) Effects of Stress

How badly a bird is affected by a certain stress will depend on several factors:

1. **Severity of the stress**. (e.g. if fighting, was the bird battered or injured?)

2. **Duration of the stress**. Being hauled in a very cramped trailer may be all right for a journey lasting an hour or two, but a three-day trip under such conditions will definitely be stressful.

3. **Individual reaction to the stress**. Some birds are much more docile than others and can handle stress a lot easier.

4. **Degree of resistance of the animal**. An animal in poor condition or with an immune system that is already weakened, will not be able to deal with stress as well as a healthy animal can.

(c) Stress Management

Being aware of what different types of situations may be stressful to emus will help a farmer to manage or avoid stress situations. Much of this is simply common sense, or will be learned sooner or later by experience. However, it is nice to be prepared before the situation arises, in order to better cope with it.

Here are some examples:

STRESS SITUATION	MANAGEMENT
1. Severe fighting	Separate fighting birds
2. Cannibalism (birds pecking on each other - occurs especially in cramped quarters or after long periods of confinement, e.g. due to bad weather)	Separate larger chicks from smaller; provide bright, colorful toys which cannot be swallowed to keep birds busy if they have to be confined inside; turn off lights; allow birds access to larger, outside pen with vegetation.
3. Heavy traffic (including people)	Remove any birds that seem to be bothered by this to a more secluded pen, or put up visual barriers.
4. Severe heat, causing birds to stand around and pant a lot.	Provide shade (trees are best); hose birds down or place sprinkler in pen.
5. Extreme cold	Provide shelters and heat lamps or heaters which are SAFE.
6. Stinging/biting insects	Fogging around pens; burn old hay around pens (smoke keeps insects at bay); apply a SAFE insect repellant to birds' heads and necks (be very careful of eyes.) Close up chicks at night if necessary, preferably **without** lights which will attract insects, or with "bug light" in a safe place. Keep standing water and manure to a minimum so insects can't breed.
7. Harassment by dogs or other predators	Electric fence around pens; shotgun; security light; radio turned on by pens at night.
8. Illness/infection	Try to determine cause and treat with appropriate medication. If necessary, tube-feed bird as described in **Section 14.10.**

(d) Prevention of stress.

Good management is the key to stress prevention. One of the most important factors in any type of livestock farming is ROUTINE. Feeding at a set time or times every day, moving quietly among the birds, collecting eggs while birds are eating or at night with a flashlight, are all sound management practices which help to keep the birds calm, docile, and used to human beings. It is also important to keep fresh water available at all times; to make any feed changes gradually; and to provide adequate space and vegetation in the pens to give the birds sufficient exercise and keep them from boredom. Larger pens with flocks of emus should contain some trees or brush, not only for shade, shelter and variety of diet, but also to provide visual barriers (screens) behind which a bird that is being chased can escape. Generally, once an aggressive emu can no longer see his quarry, he will lose interest in chasing and walk off to do something else.

It is worth noting that very young chicks are the most susceptible to HEAT STRESS, not only because their thermoregulatory system is still immature but also because they may not yet have learned through experience to move out of the hot sun into shade when necessary. If a young chick is found gasping for breath, hot to the touch and with very red skin in full sunlight - in extreme cases unable to get up - drastic action must be taken and the chick should immediately be plunged into cool water or hosed down. This will cool the chick quickly - hopefully before too much damage has been done. Using cool water rather than ice-cold will constitute less of a shock to the chick's system. In an extreme case, the chick may go into convulsions and die, not because of the cold water but rather because its temperature had already climbed too high and caused irreparable damage.

Death from heat stress is also seen occasionally in chicks hatching or about to hatch, if the temperature in the hatcher is running too high. The combination of very high temperature with an increase in the chick's body temperature as he struggles to free himself from the egg is probably what causes this. Moreover, a healthy chick that is removed from the hatcher and placed in a small box with a heat lamp is also likely to die from heat stress, if there is nowhere to get away from the source of heat. Heat lamps can raise the temperature a lot more than one realizes, and caution should always be exercised when using them.

(e) Stress and nutrition

Stress can have two bad effects on nutrition. Firstly, the bird's food intake may be reduced, as stressed birds are often too keyed-up (or depressed) to eat. Secondly, the stress itself (especially if due to infection) may cause malabsorption or an inadequate uptake of nutrients by the gut system. In short, food is not utilized properly by the bird's body. In either or both cases, this may set up a nutritional deficiency, not as a direct result of the bird's diet, but as a result of the stress affecting its food uptake. On "borderline deficient" diets, stress may be the factor to "tip the balance" and cause enough of a deficiency to produce deformities in growing chicks.

(f) Treatment of stress: Support Therapy

There will always be situations in which stress does occur, no matter how many preventive measures the farmer takes. Each such situation should of course be assessed individually, but there are a few things that can be done as support therapy for almost any bird that has suffered any kind of severe stress.

These include:

- **Rehydration** - if bird will not drink and has not had water for more than one day, the bird can be tubed (see **Section 14.10**) with water containing electrolytes (poultry vitamins/electrolytes or electrolyte solutions such as Gatorade or Pedialyte.) In extreme cases of dehydration, Lactated Ringer's Solution can be injected in fairly large quantities under the skin.

- **Energy** - glucose or dextrose, which can be absorbed directly by the gut without needing any further digestion, will provide the bird with an instant source of energy. This will raise the bird's blood sugar level if it was dangerously low, and is especially important in a very debilitated bird with little strength or energy. The glucose may be dissolved in the water/electrolyte solution used to rehydrate the bird.

- **Vitamins** - an injection of good multi-vitamins or B-12 or B-Complex will help to build up a debilitated bird, and will do no harm.

- **Probiotics** - a new word for an old remedy: Lactobacillus and related organisms, which are the "good bacteria" found in yogurt and milk curds. Yogurt, or commercial probiotics (can be purchased through feed stores or veterinary suppliers) can be tube-fed if the bird is not eating, ensuring growth of good bacteria in the gut which usually helps to exclude any harmful ones.

- **Antibiotics** - a severely stressed bird will usually have an immune system that is functioning at below-optimum level, rendering the bird more susceptible to disease. It is sometimes a good idea to put such birds on a broad-spectrum antibiotic .

- **Comfortable temperature** - a stressed bird should not be allowed to become chilled or overheated, but should be carefully monitored.

- **Seclusion** - provide a quiet environment that does not further stress the bird. In addition, chicks usually need the company of other chicks to feel secure, so one or two should be provided. Adult birds usually do better if left alone at first, or alone but within sight of other birds.

Adult birds that have been enclosed in a hot, stuffy trailer or that have been chased or beaten up by other birds can also suffer from heat stress, even if the results are not usually as drastic or potentially damaging as with chicks. Spraying the bird down with a water-hose or providing a sprinkler is usually greatly relished by the stressed-out, panting bird, and also tends to have a calming influence since emus enjoy wallowing in water.

If birds have been fighting and appear very stressed even after the worst offender(s) have been separated from the flock, scattering cracked corn (corn chops) throughout the pen works well as a calming agent, since the stimulus to eat provided by the highly visible corn tends to outweigh the urge to run around and fight.

Tranquilizers such as Acepromazine may be used on very stressed or injured birds, especially in order to treat or sew up wounds. However, as with the use of any drug, caution should be exercised and the situation assessed very carefully first. There are some cases where too much human interference will cause much greater stress to the bird than if he had just been left alone for a while. The emu farmer's knowledge and experience will help him to make the best judgment.

The ultimate goal in treating stress is to get the bird up on his feet, calm, and back to normal as soon as possible, as well as eating and drinking by himself. If a bird will not or cannot eat, it may be necessary eventually to TUBE-FEED him also (e.g. by mushing up the normal diet in water.) Very occasionally, a one-time shot of **steroids**, such as Dexamethasone, may be justified. This seems to help make the bird feel much better, and may even make him feel well enough to drink and eat on his own. A word of caution, however: steroids may:

1. depress the immune system, making the bird more vulnerable to disease
2. cause stomach ulcerations, especially after more than 1 dose
3. have other detrimental long-term effects not yet fully realized, e.g. on the future productivity of the bird.

(g) Stress to the egg

In the incubation of emu eggs, when conditions of temperature, air flow and humidity are not correct, the resultant stresses caused to the growing embryo can also impair uptake of nutrients or any other bodily functions, such as proper growth. Improper incubation techniques can therefore lead to problems, deformities or even death to developing chicks, basically as a result of stress greater than what the embryo in the egg could handle. Some deformities seen in chicks can therefore possibly be traced back to stress during incubation, and are not necessarily a result of poor breeder genetics or nutrition. This subject is covered in detail in **Chapter 10,** Incubation and Hatching.

14.9 OBSERVATION OF STOOL

There are actually several useful things one can learn from the droppings produced by an animal or bird. Here are some examples:

1. As an indicator of the general health of the bird
2. Samples can be used to check for intestinal parasites (e.g. worms) in birds

3. Used in nutritional experiments with birds, to test digestibility of different types of feed.

"Stool-watching" is something that should go right along with your "bird-watching". Just as you get to know what is normal **behavior** among your birds by observing them each day, you will also know what kind of **stool** is normal by daily observation. Any deviation from the normal should be regarded with a suspicious eye. The appearance of the stool will differ somewhat depending on what you are feeding, as well as what sort of vegetation your birds have access to. Even your soil can make a difference to the appearance of your birds' stool: some young growing birds, for instance, go through stages of eating large quantities of dirt, and often this sand or dirt shows up in their stool as well. For all these reasons, the best way to find out what is a "normal" stool is by the observation of your own birds. All outside influences should always be taken into context before making any quick judgments - e.g. effect of feed changes, medication of birds, stress to the birds etc.

It is important to remember that birds have only ONE opening or "vent" through which to pass both stool and urates (the pasty white excretory product which is birds' equivalent of urine). Also, the same opening is used by laying hens to pass eggs. Therefore, not all "stool" is actually stool; sometimes, products of the eggshell-secreting glands may also be passed.

Here are some examples of different stool appearances and the possible reasons for them:

1. **Slushy beige stool** - generally, normal for birds on rations which are based on poultry diets or some other fairly easily digestible diets. However, if the stool looks a lot like the feed, the birds may be eating more than they need.

2. **Piles of stool/formed stool**, usually a little darker in color (dark beige/greenish beige) - generally, normal for birds on rations containing a lot of fiber and/or a lot of alfalfa, such as some high-fiber ratite pellets. However, if this kind of stool is seen in birds which normally have loose stool, make sure there is not a constipation problem and that the birds have an adequate fresh water supply. If the water trough stinks, the birds probably are not drinking enough, and it must be cleaned out and refilled. While emus are not as prone to impaction as are many other ratites, an obvious sign that something is wrong is the repeated lifting of the tail and attempt to pass stool, with nothing happening. Dosing with Metamucil or mineral oil might then be necessary.

3. **Shiny, oily stool** - to be expected after you have dosed a bird with mineral oil, either on the same day or the next day.

4. **Sandy stool** - quite common in young birds which are eating a lot of sand. Perhaps the birds need some extra grit or stones to help their digestive system, or perhaps they are a little deficient in some mineral and need a vitamin/mineral supplement with their feed.

5. **Bits of corn in stool** - If adding whole corn to the birds' diet you may be turning your money into manure, since emus do not seem very good at digesting the hard outer covering of a piece of corn, and consequently, whole corn usually passes right through, undigested. Cracked corn, on the other hand, seems to be fairly well utilized although some may still pass through into the stool. At any rate, emus seem to love it and it is a good, high-energy, heat-producing supplement during periods of very cold weather. The presence of some pieces of cracked corn in the stool is usually no cause for alarm. Most of it has usually been digested, and it will be digested more efficiently if plenty of grit/small stones are provided to help the grinding action of the gizzard.

6. **Slimy, stringy, mucus-like stool** - NOT normal, and may be a sign of an intestinal problem, such as an overgrowth of bacteria. Check your bird for signs of illness, depression, or going off his feed. Your veterinarian may recommend an antibiotic, or want to check stool samples further (e.g. take cultures)

7. **Yellow stool, or yellow flecks** - again, this can be a sign of bacterial problems; keep bird under careful surveillance and check with your vet. Can also be due to extra secretions from oviduct of hen in preparation for laying.

8. **Excessively smelly stool** - can be a result of intestinal problems, as above, but may also be related to type of feed used. Birds being fed dogfood or catfish food often produce a particularly offensive-smelling stool, which may also intensify fly problems.

9. **Very dark brown stool** - if the dark color is caused by congealed blood in the stool, there is a serious problem and the vet should be called right away. Coccidiosis can cause intestinal bleeding and subsequent blood in the stool, as can several other diseases. Many are related to very high stress factors.

10. **Fresh blood (showing up bright red) in the stool** - this should be taken very seriously, as it can be a symptom of one of the following:

- Coccidiosis (gut inflammation due to protozoan parasite)
- Severe worm infestation
- Severe enteritis caused by bacteria
- Severe enteritis caused by a virus, e.g. EEE (see Section **14.5,c**).
- Internal injury (heavy fall, crashing into solid object)
- Torn (overstretched) oviduct, e.g. in passing very large egg (less serious)
- Slight injury from rough sexing or taking rectal temperature (less serious)

11. **Watery stool/diarrhea** - if stool is very watery, the bird may be drinking but not eating adequately. Check for upper respiratory infections, which may have caused swelling or inflammation, creating enough discomfort for the bird not to want to eat; or he may have a partial impaction and need to be dosed with mineral oil. True diarrhea, caused by some kind of infective organism, will often be

accompanied by a bad smell and depression in the bird, as well as dehydration and/or emaciation if you don't catch it early enough. Good support therapy, appropriate antibiotics and/or an antidiarrheal remedy may be recommended by your vet if this is the case. Note that many birds pass very loose stools in times of stress, and go back to normal once things have settled down, without needing any medication at all. In addition, birds drink large amounts of water particularly during very hot weather, so this may also make the stool much more liquid than normal without there being any problem.

12. **Frothy stool** - is also occasionally passed by birds in times of stress. If it only happens once and the bird passes normal stool before and after, it probably is nothing to worry about.

13. **Green stool** - there can be many reasons for this, some good and some bad, as follows:

(a) Dark green stool in the newborn chick - exactly what you want. This stool should be passed within 1 to 3 days of hatching, it may be in the form of one large bowel movement or several smaller ones, but it will be a fairly large amount, fairly liquid, a nice dark-green color and will usually occur before the chick has shown any interest in eating anything. It does not normally have any odor. The chick's belly becomes considerably less distended and softer after passing this stool. It can be likened to the passing of meconium in mammals.

(b) Green (eggshell-green to emerald color) stool passed by female in the beginning of breeding season - also usually a good sign, probably extra secretions from the eggshell-secreting gland as it readies itself to receive and put the final coating on eggs before they are laid.

(c) Bright green, almost fluorescent stool in young birds showing signs of weakness/illness - is often slimy as well, and can be a sign of gut erosion as a result of a serious infection or other problem. Call your veterinarian.

14. **Eggshell pieces in stool** - this is a warning signal that an egg has broken inside the hen. It is not a common occurrence, and the hen must be kept under very careful surveillance to see that she passes all of the shell. If she resumes laying, chances are all is well.

15. **Some pigmented medications** may change the normal color of the stool.

14.10 TUBE- FEEDING

When a bird is ill and not eating or drinking, it may become necessary to tube-feed him in order to keep him alive. A sick bird needs as much fluid and nourishment as a healthy bird, and sometimes more since his reserves are being depleted by fighting off infection or toxins. The problem is that because he is so sick and weak, he does not feel like eating or drinking.

The less he eats and drinks, the less reserves he has with which to continue fighting the problem. Tube-feeding can break this vicious circle by doing for the bird what he cannot or will not do for himself, thus giving him the boost that he needs.

(a) Tube-feeding the chick

The younger the chick, the more care should be exercised when tube-feeding. Not only must handling be gentle, but any liquid be introduced in very small quantities so that it does not "overflow" the esophagus and run into the trachea before the bird has a chance to close the opening. If this happens, i.e. if a bird aspirates any quantity of fluid or food down the trachea and into the lungs, pneumonia will almost certainly result and the bird may die within the day.

Any chick younger than 3 days old should definitely not need tube-feeding. It can still exist comfortably on the nutrients provided in the yolk sac. If it is starting to dehydrate within this time, this is usually a sign of yolk sac retention (**Section 10.10**) and attempts to rehydrate by tube-feeding liquids are generally not successful in any case, since the dehydration is due to a much bigger problem. In addition, the swallowing/closure of trachea-reflex may not be completely developed yet in the very new chick. Therefore as a rule of thumb, do not tube-feed any bird that has not yet started to eat and drink on its own. It is very unlikely that a very young chick would derive any benefit from tube-feeding; if it is that weak, it may die regardless. A chick that is dehydrated as a result of excessive egg weight loss during incubation, however, can be re-hydrated with Lactated Ringer's Solution injected subcutaneously (5-10cc at a time).

The most common reason to tube-feed an older chick would be debilitation due to an infection, and chicks seem to be the most susceptible to bacterial/viral infections at about 3 weeks old. Not surprisingly, this is the time by which the yolk sac has been completely absorbed except for a nodule the size of a small pea. With it, a lot of perfectly balanced nutrients and antibodies passed on from the hen have been used up,and the chick is now more vulnerable to disease-causing bacteria and viruses. If the insect population is high, the risk is even greater since insects can act as carriers (vectors) for many diseases. An infection which is very sudden and acute can deplete the bird very quickly. Tube-feeding with the appropriate nutrients can save a bird's life.

Tube-feeding a chick should be done with a large, clean plastic syringe (10 cc to 50 cc, depending on the size of the chick and what you have available) with a cut length of plastic or surgical tube attached. The ideal feeding tube is the soft, supple kind with a rounded-off end. If there is no veterinarian available who has surgical tubing, the slightly stiffer but adequate plastic tubing can be purchased from a hardware store. Length of tube should be about the length of neck of bird to be tubed.

If you have no assistant to hold the bird, gently place it in a sitting position and kneel over it in such a way that you are not placing any weight on it, but it cannot get up. Open the bird's beak and grasp the top of it firmly with your thumb and forefinger. One of the fingers can also be used to hold the bird's beak open, leaving the other hand free to slide the feeding tube down the esophagus and administer the fluid. The bird will try to pull backwards, but your hold on its beak as well as your body behind it, preventing it from getting out between your legs, should keep it in position. Larger chicks can be tube-fed in the normal standing positon.

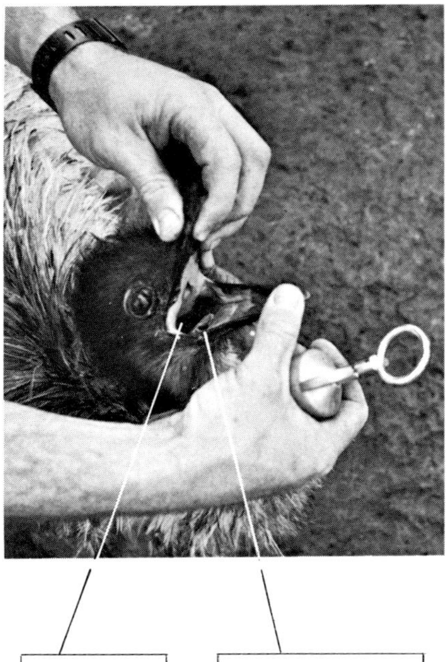

Plate 14.6 - Oesophagus is the large space at the back of the bird's mouth, windpipe the small hole at the front - it can be seen to enlarge and contract as the bird breathes. (Holes in top of beak are the inner nasal openings.)

Take the size of the bird into account when tube-feeding, and do not overfill the esophagus or administer fluid too forcefully. In chicks especially, small doses given often is much better than large doses far apart. If fluid appears to be remaining in the back of the esophagus and not going down, withdraw the tube and wait at least an hour before giving any more.

The tube should be gently inserted as far down the esophagus as possible. This reduces the risk of getting fluid into the trachea by mistake, especially if the bird struggles. Extending the neck at an upward angle and holding it extended while stroking gently underneath after the tube is withdrawn, should also help get the fluid down. Some birds will lean forward and "throw up" all the fluid as soon as the tube is removed, especially if the neck was not first held and stroked and the bird allowed to calm down. Aspiration of fluids can also occur when the bird throws up, so it is better to try and prevent this from occurring.

The photograph, **Plate 14.6**, shows clearly where the opening of the trachea is in the bird's mouth. It is also seen to flutter open and shut as the bird breathes. The remaining opening at the back of the bird's mouth is the esophagus, so the feeding tube can be inserted anywhere down it. Inserting it down one side is usually the easiest, and the opening of the trachea is also not so easily touched in this way, ensuring greater comfort and safety for the bird.

(b) Tube-feeding the adult bird

The adult bird can be tube-fed in either the sitting or standing position. If he is very sick and sitting already, this is probably the easiest, although he may raise up to squat on his hocks when the tube is inserted. In all other cases, the bird is held by one person as shown in **Fig. 3.1**, **Chapter 3,** and the tube-feeding is done by a second person. A calf-dosing syringe can be used, with or without a piece of surgical tubing attached to its end. The esophagus is very elastic and pliable, but even so, if the syringe is used without the soft tubing attached, care must be taken to hold the bird's head as still as possible, to avoid possible injury to the bird. As with chicks, insert the tube well down past the opening of the trachea, hold the neck extended and stroke it to promote swallowing, if necessary.

The main difference between tube-feeding adults and chicks is that adults can be given much larger doses at a time. Give about 100-200cc at a time, withdrawing the tube in between to allow the bird to swallow if need be. A total dose of about 500-1000cc can be given in this way to an adult bird. Once to twice a day is usually sufficient, depending on the condition of the bird. The advantage of giving larger amounts less often to adult birds is that handling can be stressful and should be minimized as far as is possible.

14.11 COLLECTING BLOOD

The best place to take blood from an emu, whether adult or chick, is in the right jugular vein. This is a vein in the top part of the neck, as shown in **Plate 14.7**. In many birds, the right jugular vein is much more prominent than the left, and the emu is no exception. The vein is usually clearly visible under the skin and can also be felt. It is about the thickness of a man's finger.

To collect blood from the adult, the standing position is recommended. This is much less stressful than forcing the bird down to the ground and restraining him there. One person holds the bird in the normal way (as outlined in **Section 3.1**) and the other finds the vein and, holding the bird's head gently to prevent struggling, inserts the needle upward and withdraws blood into the syringe. Blood flow is sometimes sluggish, but by working quietly and patiently with the bird, it should stand still for long enough to withdraw the amount required. Swabbing with antiseptic solution before and after inserting the needle is always a good idea. Hooding the bird should not be necessary, as he will often struggle less if he can see. Some birds panic when hooded and struggle more.

Chicks jump around a lot when handled, and since they are also smaller, the risk of accidentally stabbing a chick with the syringe when attempting to draw blood is greater. The best method for chicks is to lay the chick on its side or across one's lap, holding the feet together at the ankles and holding the body, while the assistant holds the head and draws blood from the jugular as before. He may raise the head and neck a little in order to accomplish this.

Blood samples may be required for pre- and post-vaccination testing as well as many other diagnostic procedures. Normal serum values for both emus and ostriches have been documented (J. Jensen, K. Hicks and E. Westerman, 1990, Texas A&M University).

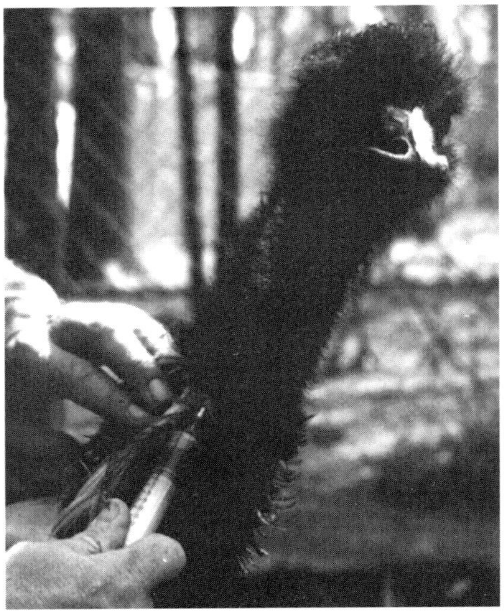

Plate 14.7(a) - Drawing blood from jugular vein using normal syringe.

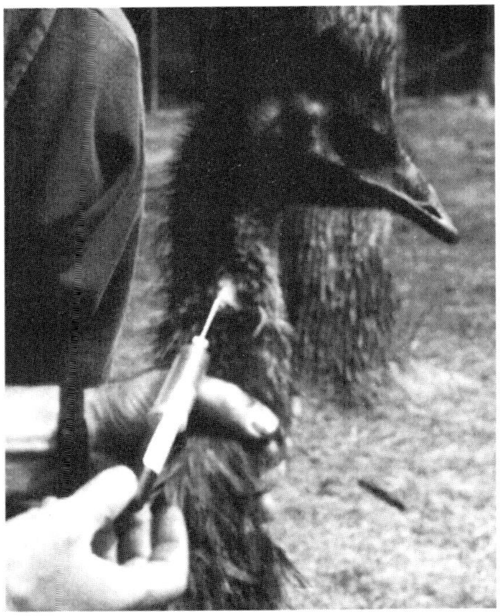

Plate 14.7(b) - Drawing blood directly into collection container.

Fig 14.1 - Emu - External Features

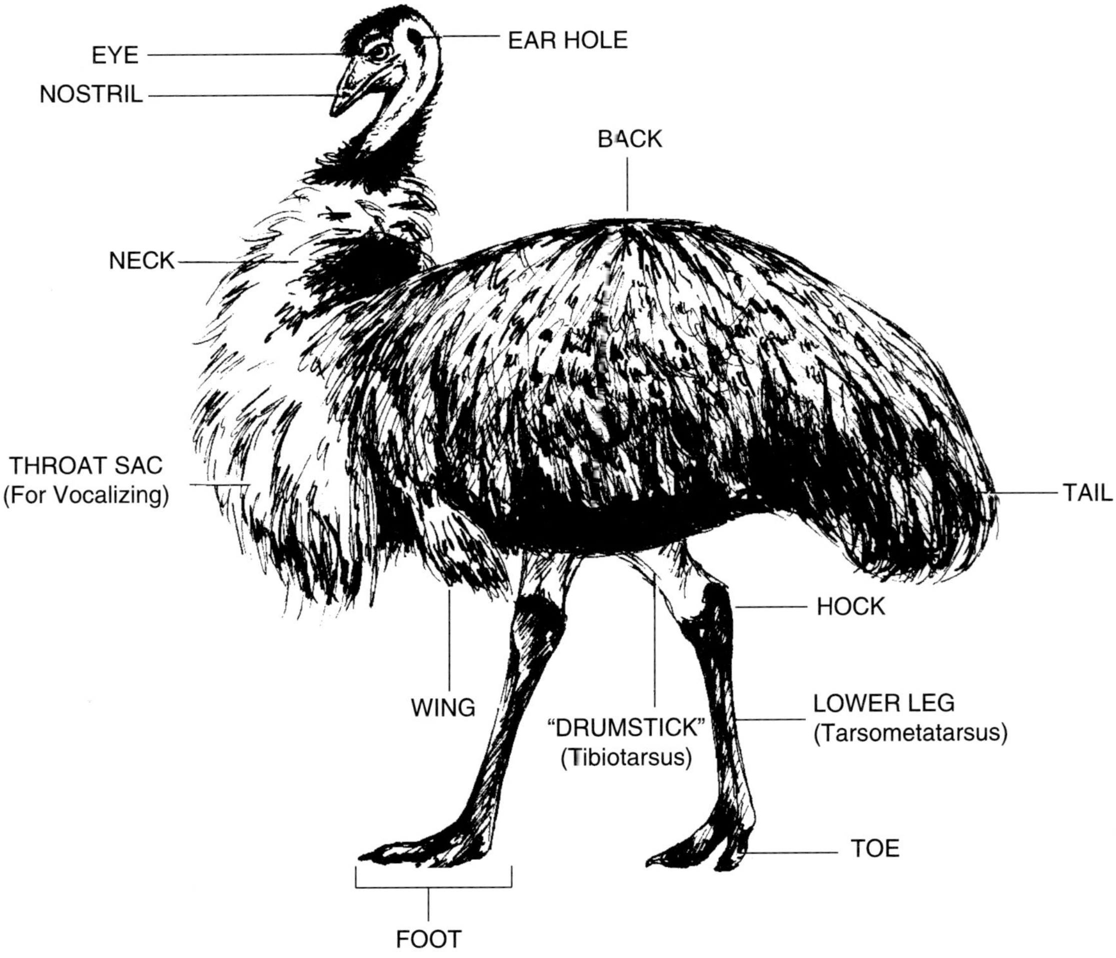

CHAPTER 15

Processing

The processing phase of commercial emu farming is just as important as any other part of emu farming because without this phase there would not be a reason to farm emus commercially. This chapter will outline how the emu farmer would process a bird that has died or that he has slaughtered for his own use. Recommendations are given on how to prepare the different products for further processing, whether for personal use or for sale.

15.1 PROCESSING METHODS

The most important part of the slaughter process is to kill the bird quickly and humanely, and to "bleed" the bird properly to ensure good taste and quality of the meat. The bird's neck is severed below the head. The severing of the jugular veins ensures that blood pumps out of the body as quickly as possible, and the carcass should be hung upside-down as soon as possible to ensure good draining of all the blood before it starts to coagulate, which would ruin the taste of the meat. Normally the nerves will cause the carcass to thrash around for a while after slaughter, as is normal in chickens, so care should be taken to avoid anyone getting kicked.

The carcass is hung by the legs, and may now be plucked of all its feathers. Clean, good quality feathers can be plucked by the handful and placed in bags according to size for sale to makers of feather jewelry and capes. Dirty or poor-quality feathers are usually discarded. The plucked carcass is now washed with clean water, and the processor should also wash his hands.

Skinning is the next step, and the initial cuts are made in the hide as shown in **Fig. 15.1(a)**. The hide and feathers around the cloaca are usually removed completely to avoid contamination of the meat. As far as possible, the processor should not touch the meat with the hand that holds the hide, since this could also cause contamination and a bad taste to the meat. If it becomes necessary to touch the meat with the (left) hand that holds the hide, wash hands first. Once the initial cuts have been made, the hide can almost totally be pulled off by hand. By pulling the hide away from the body with the left hand and pushing underneath with the right hand (using thumb or fist) in downward motions, the hide will soon be removed without any cuts, and without the extra layers of membrane or fat on its inside often caused by the use of a skinning knife. The skin is usually the tightest over the back, and here it may sometimes be necessary to carefully use a knife. The hide can be pulled down over the small wings, basically turning them inside out.

Removal of the fat layer now follows, and this is similar to a second skinning procedure. Wash hands again and remove fat. The fat is thickest on the back of the bird, and is removed by pulling with one hand while cutting it away from the carcass with the other. Wash the fat thoroughly with water, then place it in a large clean bowl or bucket.

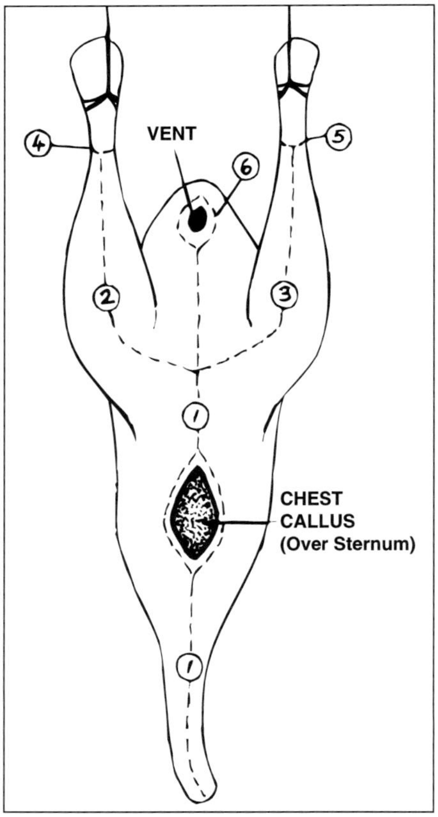

Fig. 15.1(a) - Incisions to make when skinning an emu. Ventral view.

The meat can now be removed from the carcass. All the meat from the back and top of pelvis is cut off first. Then the neck is removed. If liver and gizzard are to be used, this can be done next, being careful not to contaminate the liver with bile from the gall bladder. The ventral position of both liver and gizzard makes their removal easy. The carcass has no breast meat to speak of, so all that remains are the drumsticks and thighs. These can be separated from the carcass by cutting at the hip joints, and the carcass is allowed to drop into a bag for disposal. Separate the femurs from the drumsticks by cutting at the knee joints. The meat can now be refrigerated or processed further into roasts, de-boned meat, ground meat etc. Bones not used can later be ground up for bone meal.

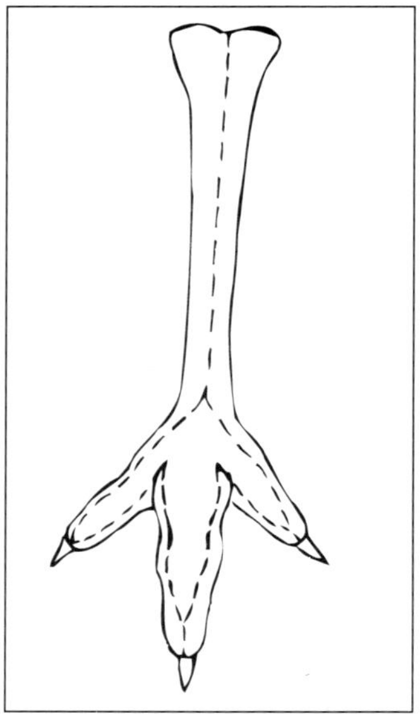

Fig. 15.1 (b) - Incisions for removal of leg skin. View: Back of leg and bottom of foot.

The lower legs from hock to foot are usually cut off from drumsticks prior to hanging the carcass. The attractive pattern of scales on the leg skins, similar to reptilian leather, makes skinning the lower legs worthwhile also. The leg skins are removed as shown in **Fig. 15.1(b)**. Split down the center of the back of the leg down to the foot and along both sides of each toe as shown, thus cutting out the thick sole pad. The hide can then be pulled off.

Both body hide and leg skins can now be checked for any fat deposits left during skinning, and cleaned off if need be by scraping. Wash the body hide with water to remove blood or dirt, and spread it open flat on a clean surface with the inside up. Salt it liberally, using about a can of table salt (1 lb) or the same amount of coarse salt. Pour salt into middle of hide and spread with the hands all the way to the edges of the skin so that all of it is covered. Allow it to dry for 3 - 7 days. When dry, roll up the hide loosely and gently (do not fold) and send to the tanner. This dry-salting procedure preserves the skin for several months, provided it is not allowed to get wet again.

If tanning can be done immediately, skin can merely be refrigerated after washing. Skins should not be frozen, as water expands when it freezes and so any ice crystals forming in the skin will cause damage.

The fat may now be cut up into small pieces or even run through a meat grinder. Water is added to it to begin with, and it is rendered by boiling for a long time, in a large stainless-steel pot, with oil being poured off at intervals as it floats to the top. The oil is poured into open glass containers and allowed to cool. Rendering is continued until all the fat is cooked away to crisp remnants. The oil can be filtered or skimmed if there are any visible impurities, and as it separates on cooling into a semi-solid portion and a clear oil, it can be poured off again if so desired. The oil can then be sent to buyers or manufacturers.

Microwaving is also a possible method of rendering oil, and there may be some commercial methods as well. Plastic containers are generally not used for storage of emu oil as it appears to seep through them and make the outsides greasy.

Note: The meat of a bird that has died, whether from known or unknown causes, should not be used for human consumption. Not only was the bird not bled so that the meat will probably have a bad taste, but also there could already be bacteria or toxins in the tissues. The bird may, however, be processed for its other products (leather, oil, feathers). A bird that has broken its leg and needs to be put down can be used for meat, since the normal slaughter process will be used.

15.2 "BLOWING" THE INFERTILE EGG

Since emu eggs make rather attractive ornaments, whether displayed in their natural state or carved/etched/painted, it is worth the time and effort to learn good techniques of emptying any infertile eggs. There are egg decorating clubs and societies in many areas who will buy egg shells of all kinds in order to make clocks, jewelry boxes and many other kinds of ornaments, and emu eggs are often sought after because of their unusual color. Establishing yourself as a supplier of good-quality, clean, attractive emu eggshells can be an additional small sideline to your emu farming business.

It is **not** necessary to make two holes in an egg in order to blow out its contents. One hole is sufficient. The hole is usually made in the large end of the egg, so that the hole is hidden in its base when the egg is displayed on a stand. To make a hole that is round and even, without any cracks around it, the egg can either be drilled with an electric drill, or a Phillips screwdriver can be used, gently turning it while applying pressure until it is through the shell. The hole may be widened, if necessary, using a larger screwdriver.

Since even an infertile egg still has an inner and outer shell membrane, and since the inner shell membrane separates the egg contents from the air space in the egg, it is necessary to put the screwdriver all the way into the egg to its bottom in order to poke a hole through this membrane and allow the egg contents to escape. (In a "tinny"-sounding egg which has been shaken until it sloshes, the membrane has already been broken.)

While the contents of the egg may now be shaken out by hand, and the egg then rinsed and shaken out again repeatedly, this is a very tedious process. The quicker way of emptying and cleaning the egg is to use one of the following two methods:

1. Using a length of flexible plastic or surgical tubing, available at hardware stores or vet supply stores, insert the tubing through the hole into the egg and run water through it. The pressure of the water coming in will force the egg contents out of the same hole, provided there is a little space between the tubing and the edges of the hole. Continue until the only thing coming out of the egg is clean water. Blowing air into the egg via the tube also works, but is more tedious.

2. Using a can of WD-40 oil with its short, straight tube attachment, insert tube into hole as far as it will go (after first shaking the can) and squirt oil into egg. The contents of the egg will again be forced out, under pressure, usually fairly quickly. Note: using WD-40 on an egg that is rotten, may cause it to burst under the additional pressure. Handle rotten eggs gently and carefully so as to avoid any such unpleasant experiences, or do not attempt to "blow" rotten eggs at all.

Many infertile eggs have no unpleasant smell at all as they were not invaded by bacteria at any time. Nevertheless, it is a good practice to disinfect every blown-out egg with a solution of liquid bleach and water (several tablespoons to a gallon) or some other good disinfectant. The advantage of using bleach is of course that it is cheap, readily available and extremely effective against smells of all kinds since it kills both bacteria and most fungi. As a final step, rinse the egg (using the flexible tubing) several times with this mixture. Shake it out, and place it on a curtain ring with paper towel underneath it to drain and dry.

To disinfect several eggs at the same time, some people will prepare the bleach-mixture in a bucket and immerse all the eggs in it, making sure to hold each egg under-water for long enough to fill it up completely. Eggs should not be left too long in such a mixture since the bleach will begin to etch into the surface of the egg, whitening it. This can, of course, be an interesting effect also for decorative purposes. The light green areas of the egg will whiten first, while the dark green turns duller, giving a very mottled effect.

Emu eggs usually turn darker with age, some becoming almost black.

Egg Art

Painting - Eggs may be painted with either oil paint or acrylic paint. The acrylic dries a lot quicker but will have a dull finish versus the shinier finish of oil paint. Acrylic paint can, however, be given a shiny finish by the application of clear enamel paint, clear nail varnish or clear decoupage glaze, applied once the paint has dried. This helps preserve and protect the finished picture.

Etching - Because the emu egg is made up of several layers (going lighter green towards the inside, with the innermost layer being white) the egg can be etched to achieve a cameo-type effect, carving deeper for the lighter colors. Australian Aborigines are experts at this, and many carve by hand, using a knife or hand-held blade. A Dremmel tool with various bits may also be used. For fine work, a dentist's drill is suitable.

Carving - Using a good dentist's drill, the carving of patterns all the way through the shell is possible without breaking or cracking the shell. While it may take some time (and broken eggs) to become an expert at this, the results are rewarding. Emu eggs carved in this way may even be used as lamps, since the carved patterns will allow light through the otherwise opaque shell. A dentist's drill is also useful for cutting an egg in half (usually lengthwise) in order to make a jewelry box, or for cutting doors or windows into eggs. Special glues, hinges and decorative items made specifically for eggs are available through egg decorating clubs and societies.

REFERENCES

1. McLelland, J. 1991. A Color Atlas of Avian Anatomy. Wolfe Publishing Ltd., England.

2. Mönnig, H.O. and Veldman, F.J. 1989. Handbook on Stock Diseases, Fourth Revised Edition. Tafelberg Publishers Ltd, Cape Town, South Africa.

3. Jordan, Rick. 1989. Parrot Incubation Procedures. Silvio Mattacchione and Co., Pickering, Ontario (Canada).

4. Maynard, Leonard A. and Loosli, John K. 1969. Animal Nutrition, Sixth Edition. McGraw-Hill, Inc. New York.

5. National Research Council Subcommittee on Poultry Nutrition. 1984. Nutrient Requirements of Poultry, Eighth Revised Edition. National Academy Press, Washington, D.C.

6. Hoyt, D.F. 1979. Practical methods of estimating volume and fresh weight of bird eggs. Auk, 96, 73-77.

ACKNOWLEDGEMENTS

It would take a whole volume to fully acknowledge all those who have in some way contributed towards the making of this book by their input, encouragement and support. Without the hard work and dedication of these numerous individuals - emu farmers, veterinarians and many others whom we are privileged to call our friends - the emu industry would not be where it is today.

To all of you, our thanks.